KU-592-764

Judith **Dwyer**
Zhanming **Liang**
Valerie **Thiessen**
Angelita **Martini**

2ND EDITION

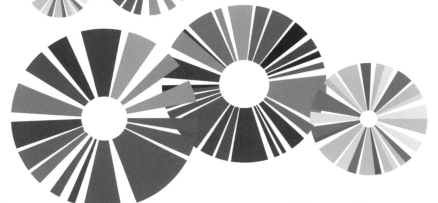

Project Management
in Health and Community Services

Getting good ideas to work

NEWMAN UNIVERSITY
BARTLEY GREEN
BIRMINGHAM B32 3NT

CLASS 362 1068
BARCODE 01674072
AUTHOR Dwy

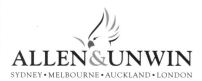

ALLEN&UNWIN
SYDNEY • MELBOURNE • AUCKLAND • LONDON

First published in 2004
This edition published in 2013

Copyright © Judith Dwyer, Zhanming Liang, Valerie Thiessen and Angelita Martini 2013

All rights reserved. No part of this book may be reproduced or transmitted in
any form or by any means, electronic or mechanical, including photocopying,
recording or by any information storage and retrieval system, without prior
permission in writing from the publisher. The Australian *Copyright Act 1968*
(the Act) allows a maximum of one chapter or 10 per cent of this book, whichever
is the greater, to be photocopied by any educational institution for its educational
purposes provided that the educational institution (or body that administers it) has
given a remuneration notice to Copyright Agency Limited (CAL) under the Act.

Allen & Unwin
83 Alexander Street
Crows Nest NSW 2065
Australia

Phone: (61 2) 8425 0100
Email: info@allenandunwin.com
Web: www.allenandunwin.com

Cataloguing-in-Publication details are available
from the National Library of Australia
www.trove.nla.gov.au

ISBN 978 1 74331 048 9

Set in 11.5/14 pt Bembo by Midland Typesetters, Australia

Printed by Hang Tai Printing Company Ltd

10 9 8 7 6 5 4 3 2 1

WITHDRAWN

Project
Management
in Health and
Community Services

N 0167407 2

Contents

Glossary of terms

80 hour rule   A rough guideline about the normal scale of activities in a work breakdown structure: no single activity should require more than 80 hours (or two weeks) of work.

Activities   A collection of related tasks that contribute to a single deliverable.

Benefits realisation   A method of evaluating project success according to whether the intended benefits (financial or other) are achieved, often some time after the project itself is completed. Used most frequently in information systems projects.

Best practice   A method or technique that has consistently shown results superior to those achieved with other means which may be used as a benchmark.

Budget   A financial document that forecasts or plans the expected dollar inflows (revenue) and dollar outflows (expenses) for a project.

Business case   A document that describes an intended service or 'business' in operational and financial terms, and seeks to establish that the service as planned can be financially viable (or profitable)—a positive business case is one in which the revenue/benefits outweigh the costs.

Buy-in   The level of support among any group of stakeholders (often staff and management) for the project and/or the proposed changes.

Cash flow   The movement of money into and out of a business, project or financial entity during a specified period of time.

Close/close-out   The fourth phase of the project cycle when the process of handover, or transitioning from the project to the new method or state, is completed.

Commissioning   This term has two meanings:
1. The process of ensuring that a new facility, piece of equipment or service is fully operational.
2. The process of engaging a team, company or consultant to conduct a project, service or other activity on behalf of the funding agency.

Contingency   A potential problem or change in the project; an amount of money or other resource held within the project to cover elements of risk or uncertainty.

Control   Ensuring that the project keeps to the agreed project scope, budget, schedule and quality.

Cost-benefit analysis (CBA)   Estimates (in monetary terms) the costs and benefits (or measure of effect) of an intervention or program.

Cost-effectiveness analysis (CEA)   Compares relative cost and outcomes (or effect) of two or more interventions with the effect expressed in non-monetary terms using 'natural units' such as cure rate or reduction in the incidence of a disease.

Cost-utility analysis (CUA)   Expresses outcomes in the non–monetary unit of quality adjusted life years (QALYs) so that comparisons of benefit can be made between alternative treatments or interventions.

Critical success factors (CSF)   The important aspects of projects (and their contexts) that are known to affect the achievement of outcomes.

Deliverable leg   A graphical presentation in a WBS of the work required to complete each deliverable.

Deliverables   The concrete goods or services that will be produced by the project and handed over on its completion.

Direct costs   The costs incurred by and for the project that would not otherwise be incurred by the organisation.

Economic evaluation   Type of analysis that estimates the relative value of alternative options.

Effectiveness   The extent to which planned outcomes are achieved by a service or product in normal conditions (rather than in the laboratory or in trials). The answer to the question 'does it work in practice?'.

Efficacy   The extent to which planned outcomes are achieved by a service or product in ideal conditions. The answer to the question 'can it work?'.

Escalate　Taking problems or issue/s higher in the organisation in order for them to be resolved, or implementing the next level of action required to overcome an identified risk.

Evaluation indicators　Markers of a project's progress, change and success.

Evidence-based practice　Decisions in (clinical) practice based on evidence from research studies and other sources of reliable information (for example, internal data).

Exclusions　What is out of the project scope (what the project won't do).

Expenditure items　Expenses incurred by a project.

Feasibility study　A process that objectively and rationally examines whether a proposed project, service or system can be successfully implemented.

Gantt chart　A commonly used method of presenting the timelines and tasks of a project, and of charting actual progress. It plots activities (in rows) against the timeline (in columns), thus showing the relationships between them.

Gap analysis　An assessment of information about gaps and potential capacity in the available service system.

Go/no go　The time at which the organisation decides whether or not to proceed with the next stage of a project, or to accept a chosen system or model.

Go-live　The time at which a product, deliverable or outcome is put into practice.

Goal　A statement of what the project aims to achieve.

Grey literature　Research that is unpublished or not published in the peer-reviewed research literature, such as government reports and policy documents.

Impact evaluation　Measures achievement of the project's goals and objectives—that is, it focuses on the short-term results.

In-kind funding　Resources (other than money) that are provided to enable or support a project, such as staff time, office space and administrative support.

Indirect costs　Costs incurred that are not readily identified and attributed to a particular project. These costs may be necessary for the implementation and completion of the project, but are 'built in' or shared with other activities within the organisation.

Labour items Budgeted costs for staff required to do the work of the project, both those employed by the organisation and external contractors.

Lean thinking An approach to business processes (or processes of care) that aims to create more value (for patients, clients or customers) while minimising resource waste (cost, time, errors and rework).

Literature review (see also Systematic literature review) A process of finding, describing, summarising, evaluating and clarifying evidence found in the literature.

Monitor Conduct regular review and reporting of the project progress.

Needs assessment or needs analysis An activity to develop a comprehensive understanding of a problem or need in the community or population, in order to identify interventions or strategies that can solve those problems and address those needs.

Objectives Statements of the steps or changes that need to be achieved in order to achieve the goal.

Outcome evaluation Measures the longer term achievements or results of the project.

Probity (tender process integrity) A tendering process that is fair, impartial, transparent, secure, confidential and compliant with legislative obligations and government policy.

Process evaluation Measures the effectiveness of the strategies and methods used in the project, and the skill of their execution.

Program A group of projects managed in a coordinated way; or a service, intervention or set of activities that aims to meet a health or social care need.

Program evaluation and review technique (PERT) A statistical tool for scheduling projects which specifies and analyses the tasks involved and significant milestones.

Program logic A method of planning and evaluating projects that specifies the links between the goals of a service or project and the inputs, processes, outputs and impacts/outcomes it will produce to achieve those goals.

Project concept brief/proposal A short document that outlines the rationale, goals and scope of a project, prepared for the purposes of seeking early in-principle support for a project idea.

Project/s director Title used sometimes for the leader of a single large project, but often for a member of the organisation's executive or senior management team who has responsibility for strategy and innovation, including leading a group of projects.

Project life cycle   A framework of the phases that projects must move through in order to progress from 'a good idea' to completion.

Project management   The methods by which those responsible for a project make it happen and monitor and control the time, cost and quality of projects.

Project manager   The person responsible for managing the whole project, across the various departments and staff who may be needed.

Project portfolio   The collection of projects being conducted by the organisation, or by major divisions within it.

Project triangle   The three dimensions that define the project: quality (or specifications), time and resources.

Scope   The reach and boundaries of the project—'who, what, where, when and how'—within defined limits.

Scope creep   Unmanaged changes to scope—usually expansion.

Sign-off   Formal approval.

Soft projects   Complex undertakings aimed at intangible results.

Sponsor   The executive who manages, administers, monitors, funds and is responsible for the overall project delivery.

Stage   A distinct part of a large project with its own outputs or deliverables; stages are often separated by decision-points.

Stakeholders   Individuals and organisations actively involved in the project, or whose interests may be affected as a result of the project, or who may exert influence over the project and its results.

Status report   Advice to the steering committee, project sponsor and other stakeholders as to whether the project is on track to deliver the planned outcomes, and to highlight where their decision-making or direct help is needed.

Steering committee   A formal advisory committee of high level project stakeholder representatives and/or experts, normally chaired by the project sponsor, that provides guidance on key issues, acts as the decision-making body for large changes to the project during its life, authorises acceptance of reports and deliverables and acts as a sounding board for the project team.

Systematic literature review (see also Literature review)   The review of literature focusing on a specific research question. The process includes identifying, appraising, selecting and synthesising all high-quality research evidence relevant to that question.

Tender   An offer submitted by interested bidders (organisations that apply or 'bid' to win the contract) to the agency commissioning the project (sometimes called the 'purchaser').

Tracking   Monitoring the progress of the project by determining how and when activities and milestones need to be reviewed.

Variance(s)   A measurable change from a known standard or baseline—the difference between what is expected and what is actually accomplished.

Work breakdown structure (WBS)   A tool that the project team uses to plan the strategies, activities and tasks required to achieve the deliverables (and the goal) of the project. WBS enables detailed planning of the work, budget and timeline required for the project.

Work package   All scheduled activities and tasks (with milestones) required to complete a deliverable in a WBS.

List of figures, tables and cases

Figures

Tables

Cases

About the authors

Professor Judith Dwyer is the Director of Research for the Department of Health Care Management in the Flinders University School of Medicine, and is a former CEO of Southern Health Care Network in Melbourne, and of Flinders Medical Centre in Adelaide. She is a Research Program Leader for the Lowitja Institute, Australia's national Aboriginal health research institute, and teaches in the Flinders University Masters of Health Administration. She is currently Deputy Chair of the board of the Cancer Council, South Australia. Her research interests include the governance of the Australian health system, and Aboriginal health services and policy.

Dr Zhanming Liang is a Senior Lecturer in health service management in the School of Public Health and Human Biosciences at La Trobe University in Melbourne. She developed her experience in planning and evaluation and health service management before joining academia. Her current research interests include management competency, competence assessment for health service managers, and evidence-informed decision-making in health service management. Her teaching responsibilities include project management, planning and evaluation, health care quality, and the Australian health system. She is currently a Director of DRUG-ARM Australasian Board and Book Review Editor of the *Australian Journal of Primary Health*.

Ms Valerie Thiessen is the Director of IT Projects and Business Applications at Northern Health in Melbourne, and holds qualifications in health information management, health services management and project management. Her experience includes roles in health information, business management, project management and consulting roles in both the private and public sectors in Australia. More recently, Valerie has been involved in and consulted on a variety of projects including clinical, radiology and patient information system implementations.

Dr Angelita Martini is a Senior Research Fellow in the Department of Health Care Management at Flinders University in South Australia. Her current research is focused on governance of first people's health systems and organisations, and models of care in cancer services. She currently coordinates the doctoral program and teaches in the Masters of Health Administration. Dr Martini was formerly a Senior Lecturer in public health, medicine and Aboriginal health.

Acknowledgements

We owe a particular debt of gratitude to our colleague Professor Pauline Stanton, Head of the School of Management and Information Systems at Victoria University, Melbourne. Professor Stanton was one of the authors of the first edition, and made a vital contribution to the development of the thinking on which this book is based.

We are also indebted to the anonymous people who were interviewed for the research that informs the book. We thank them for their generosity, honesty and insights into their own experiences of projects and project management, and their analysis of the role of projects in the health and community services sector.

We would like to thank several friends and colleagues who helped us with ideas, support, stories and resources, including Barbara Allen, John Anderson, Jason Cloonan, Mark Cormack, Henk de Deugd, Christine Fuller, Michele Herriot, Peter Howard, Catherine James, Kathryn Kenny, Margot Mains, Jackie McLeod, Alison McMillan, Gregg Ryan, Steve Walker and Paul Zadow. Finally, our thanks go to Lee Koh and Liudi Xia for editorial and literature searching assistance.

Introduction

Writing a book is a project too. This second edition came about because there is still a need in health and community services for project management approaches that are tailored to the sector. In completing this project, we had many discussions about our own experience as project managers and felt confident that a book that drew on the richness of the industry—and told the stories of the challenges, dilemmas and successes of the people within it—had much to offer.

This good idea then had to go through the many stages of definition and redefinition, planning and implementation, always under pressure of time. We read the literature, we interviewed people active in project leadership and project management, and talked the project over with colleagues, friends and loved ones. We also wrote a plan, divided up the work, committed to deadlines and struggled to meet them. The plan was revisited more than once, some tasks were swapped around, and the business of integrating all our contributions to make sure that the whole was more than the sum of its parts was an important challenge.

There are features of this edition that we think will work better for readers who need a guide as they struggle with their projects (or their project portfolios), as well as for those who are studying project management, or funding and commissioning projects. But some things don't change. Managing people is still one of the most difficult parts of the project management process, a problem that is not limited to the health and community services industry, but which does have a particular shape and flavour in this complex, people-rich environment.

Managing change is also a continuing challenge. Old ways of funding, administering and managing health and community care were swept away in a great wave of change in the last two decades of the twentieth century, and the pace of change has only increased since.

Managers, policy-makers and professionals have responded with energy and creativity, finding new ways of providing care, of doing business and of implementing and sustaining change. Real sustained gains in effectiveness and productivity have been made. But at the same time, it has proven difficult to bring new methods into practice, to learn from research and to change old habits and ways of thinking. The approach and methods of project management have a rich contribution to make as people, professions and agencies continue to search for effective ways to innovate, change and grow.

This book seeks to address a growing need in the health and community services sector for concise and critical guidance in the use of projects: when to use the project approach, how to design projects for success and how to choose among the many methods and tools. The need for guidance is growing because more and more of what needs to be done in the sector is being conceived of, funded and managed as projects—while most of the literature on project management is designed for the engineering, IT or manufacturing industries. We aim to provide the information and the analytical framework that organisations, managers and project managers require in order to run successful projects, for the right outcomes, in a way that enhances the overarching purpose or strategy of their organisations.

How to use this book

The book can be read from start to finish for an experience of immersion in the world of projects and project management. Or parts can be used as a reference and guide by project managers at various stages of their work. Senior managers and the providers of funding for projects might use it to enhance their appreciation of what their project ideas might actually entail, and to support their decision-making about which project proposals to fund or approve.

Chapter 1 explains the basics, and provides a model for thinking about project success and failure. It also outlines the research we conducted for this edition. Chapter 2 addresses the context of health and community services, and the factors that assist organisations to be successful in their project work. It suggests criteria that both senior managers and funders of projects could use to assist in their decision-making (and that those seeking to get their projects approved might use to improve their chances). Chapter 3 explains the project life cycle and the methods and tools of project management, and discusses the emerging career pathways for those with a talent for 'getting good ideas to work'. These three chapters establish the basis for the detailed guide to managing a project that makes up the following chapters.

Chapters 4 to 8 address the practice of project management, according to the phases of the project life cycle—initiation, planning, implementation and closure. The use of a broad range of methods, approaches and tools is explained, along with the challenge of making change happen through projects. These chapters are designed to meet the needs of both the practising project manager and those entering the field of project management. It is also essential reading for those who manage groups of projects, plan project strategy for their organisations, or lead the planning and development effort.

Throughout the book, worked examples and project stories are used to illustrate the methods and tools. We have included lots of headings and subheadings in each chapter to help the reader locate particular topics of interest, as well as understand the logical development of the material. A summary at the end of each chapter recaps the major points, and case studies and useful checklists are highlighted within the text for easy reference. Additional resources are listed at the end of each chapter.

There is a lot of technical language in the world of projects, which we seek to explain and demystify throughout. Terms that might be unfamiliar are explained in the glossary at the beginning of this book, and shown in **bold** type the first time they appear in each chapter.

We are now at the lovely moment of handover—the work has been done, celebrations have been held, and all the documentation is in order. For this project, the final evaluation will come later, and is in the hands of our readers.

1

Why project management?

This chapter explains what projects are and how projects are used by organisations, including those in health and community services. It also discusses why project management is important, and what project management can deliver. It covers the origins and development of project management as a method, and the reasons for its increasing popularity. We briefly discuss the results of research we conducted for this book, and the chapter ends with a model for success in project management in health and community services.

What is a project?

> There are those who make things happen; there are those who
> let things happen; there are those who wonder what happened.
> The project manager leads by making things happen!
>
> *(Gido & Clements 1999: 79)*

A project is a unique set of inter-related **activities** designed to produce
a set of **deliverables** and achieve a defined **goal** within clearly defined
time, cost and quality constraints (Burke 2003; Westland 2006). That
is, a project is a one-off effort, requires resources and is traditionally
described as having a '3D' objective: to meet specifications, to finish
on time and to be done within **budget** (for example, Rosenau 1998)
(see Figure 1.1). This is called the **project triangle** or 'iron triangle'
(Atkinson 1999; Westerveld 2003). A more recent definition (Roberts
2011: 12) emphasises the need for the project's benefits to outweigh the
cost of the resources invested in it.

The business of bringing together people and resources to achieve
a one-off purpose (such as building a pyramid) has been one of the
defining features of human society for as long as we can imagine.
However, **project management** tools first emerged in engineering in the early 1900s, with the projects simply being managed by the
architects, engineers and builders themselves. From the 1950s, project

Figure 1.1 The '3D' objective of a project

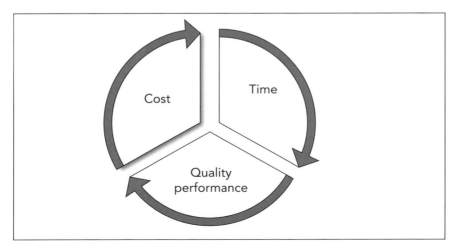

management tools and techniques were systematically applied to engineering and spread to other fields, such as construction and defence activity (Cleland & Gareis 2006). Since then, the rapid development of modern project management has seen it recognised as a distinct discipline, with two worldwide professional organisations: the International Project Management Association (IPMA), established in 1967, and the Project Management Institute (PMI), in 1969. The PMI publishes a popular project management guidebook: *A Guide to the Project Management Body of Knowledge* (PMBOK® Guide) and defines a project as:

> a temporary endeavour undertaken to create a unique product or service or result. The temporary nature of a project indicates a definite beginning and end. The end is reached when the project's objectives have been achieved or when the project is terminated because its objectives will not or cannot be met, or when the need for the project no longer exists . . . Projects can have social, economic and environmental impacts that far outlast the projects themselves.
>
> *(PMI 2008: 5)*

In the past decade, we have seen increasing attention given to projects in health and community services, and most postgraduate courses in health care management, public health and health promotion incorporate project management competencies. Projects are more common than many would believe, but are sometimes not recognised:

> . . . people do lots of projects and they do lots of improvements but they don't recognise it as such. Often projects almost sort of happen by default . . . if people recognised that what they were doing is actually an improvement project they'd actually probably do it better . . . or they would share that information more.
>
> *(Hospital clinical leader)*

Although each project is unique, they all have some common characteristics. By definition, projects are one-off efforts to achieve a goal, with a beginning and end and a budget/resources. They also have a common life cycle; have defined deliverables that are achieved and can be measured by the end of the project; and may enable changes that transform processes, performance and culture (Burke 2003; Westland 2006; Turner 2007).

Projects also have several characteristics that can make them challenging. Firstly, each project is a *unique* and novel endeavour (Oisen 1971; Westland 2006), so, by definition, it hasn't been done before. Depending on its size, it may also require the involvement of many different occupational groups, different parts of the organisation, and different functions and resources, and these must be brought together to focus on the achievement of the **objectives** of the project.

The targets set by a project are often *complex* and can require levels of technical performance not yet generally achieved in the field (Oisen 1971; Westland 2006; PMI 2008). Complexity can arise from the different perspectives of various disciplines involved, the inexperience of the players, the number of interested parties, the geographic spread, and so on. For example, hospital redevelopment projects are typically very complex undertakings involving constructing a new facility on an existing site, introducing new technology and procedures, and changing the size and structure of the staff, while also continuing to offer services. In a project such as this, important **stakeholders** may be opposed to one another, different departments with different agendas will be participating and political involvement will be high. All of these factors can have an impact on decision-making, the project **scope**, the communication challenge and the chances of success or failure.

Managing a project also represents managing a *dynamic* situation, as the unexpected is always happening, (Cleland & King 2008). When a new problem arises, it must be addressed immediately, because the project is limited by its timelines. It is expensive to change the specifications of a new IT system, for example, once design work is underway. It can be expensive in a different way to change the goals or scope of an organisational restructuring project. Senior management can dictate a change of direction to respond to changes in the internal or external environments, but doing so is likely to damage commitment and goodwill among those affected, who often value certainty. Team dynamics can also be critical when a wide range of skills and expertise is required by the project.

Managing projects can be similar to managing *high-risk* businesses (Westland 2006; Chen 2011). Projects are often used to trial new ideas, so there is a lot of uncertainty and some unknowns. For large projects, estimation of time and cost can be more an art than a science. Projects can also be at risk from external factors such as stakeholder resistance, political intervention, changes of policy direction and funding cuts.

Projects can *vary in scope* from something as simple as implementing the use of a new type of catheter to a complex undertaking like introducing a new model of care. Projects may be visible to the whole organisation and wider community—glamorous and exciting—or they may be hidden away in a small team or department—committed people doing good work.

The risks of projects are many, including the chance that they will overrun their timelines and costs. As one of the senior managers we interviewed for this book noted:

> I suppose some of it is just around taking the risk to do it. When some new projects start you can't imagine—I mean the 'smoke free' one is a good example; no-one ever thought that hospitals would be smoke free but eventually we got there so some of it's just about making a start because it seems overwhelming to get to the end result.
>
> *(Hospital clinical leader)*

The project life cycle

Although projects are highly varied in almost every characteristic, they all move through a common basic life cycle—from initiation to closing, via planning/preparation and implementation phases. Figure 1.2 shows a model of the **project life cycle** in these four phases. Thinking about the phases in a project life cycle is useful both for seeing the whole picture and for planning and managing each phase. But it would be a mistake to think that having an idea, conceptualising the idea into a project, and successfully completing the project is a linear process. Projects generally don't go exactly as planned, and **project managers** have a critical role in monitoring progress, identifying problems or variations, modifying the plan and taking action accordingly.

Although it is useful to plan and manage the project in phases, the phases are not really separate—rather, they tend to overlap and often lack clear boundaries. Even when the team is using a project management method with formal approval steps, there may not be an obvious point where they can say 'the initiation phase is complete, we are now starting

Figure 1.2 Project life cycle

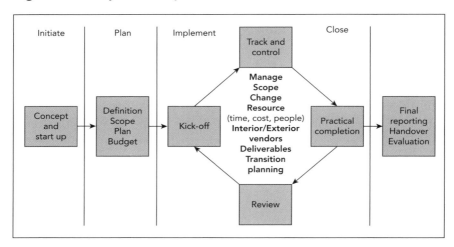

Source: Adapted from Liang (2011) and Kloppenborg (2009)

the planning phase'. Projects can also go backwards—for example, problems in the project planning can force a rethink of the original concept. The project life cycle is addressed in more detail in Chapter 3.

Projects in health and community services

The use of project management methods is well established in the health and community services industry. Staff in local government, and in community health centres, began defining much of their community development and health promotion work as projects in the 1970s and 1980s, and developed in-house templates and protocols to plan and manage their work. These methods have proven effective, and are now standard practice in the field.

Hospitals have been using project management methods for capital and IT projects for many years, but widespread application of these methods (learnt largely from contractors and consultants and sometimes from staff with community health backgrounds) to their core business only began in the 1990s. In recent years, projects have been used to introduce changes such as new care processes and service improvement. The introduction of continuous quality improvement methods and of process reengineering also provided important sources of project thinking and project skill development. Although the published research on project management in health and community services is limited, project management tools and methods are widely used, particularly to improve quality and safety and to reduce costs (Sa Couto 2008).

Government health and human service departments, on the other hand, initially tended to focus on in-house project development and approval processes and workflow management methods. More recently, there has also been an increase in the use of project management tools and software to guide project work. Many government departments are skilled users of contracted projects, and there has often been a transfer of project skills from the consultants to departmental staff. The **tendering**, **commissioning** and funding of projects in health and community services, in order to test new ideas and develop new services (in conjunction with management consultants or in-house), has been a common method of encouraging innovation, quality improvement and the move into new models of care or modes of service delivery:

> Projects are initiated at all levels of the organisation and are often in response to changing government policy, and are usually . . . service delivery driven.
>
> *(Hospital senior manager)*

In health and community services, project management methods are used for four basic purposes:

1. The development of new services, **programs** or technologies
2. To improve existing services, care processes, work practices or service delivery models
3. The implementation of new organisational structures or systems
4. The construction, acquisition and/or commissioning of new equipment and facilities.

The first three of these purposes are fundamentally about the management of change and basic organisational strategy. For success in this kind of project, change management principles should apply, and it is critical for project managers to understand the real impact of the project on themselves and other staff (Levasseur 2010). The experience of Australian hospitals in projects to improve the flow of patients through emergency departments is a good example. These projects set out to achieve change to longstanding work practices and relationships. While some of the difficulties are technical (for example, lack of good automated information systems for managing patient flow), the more significant problems arise from the need to change the roles of clinical staff, and the relationships among different medical specialties (Proudlove, et al. 2003).

Research for this book

We conducted interviews with thirteen leaders (in senior management and project management roles) in health and community service organisations in Australia for this edition of the book. We asked them about their practice in decision-making about projects, in shaping their **project portfolios** and in the use of tools and techniques, and about the reasons projects in their organisations work well or fail—and how they judge the results. We recorded and transcribed the interviews, and analysed the material to identify the major trends and ideas. And we compared these results with similar research conducted nearly ten years earlier for the first edition. The results of this research are summarised here, and presented throughout the book, along with quotes from the participants.

The participants were chosen to represent a broad range of perspectives and operational areas, from private hospitals to statutory agencies of government, from health promotion to information systems development, and those on both sides of the funding relationship (that is, funders and providers of services) in the private sector and in government. On the basis of this research, and our review of recent research in project management journals, we have concluded that the health and community services industry in Australia has changed the way it uses projects in three important ways: there is more attention given to managing an organisation's investment in projects as a portfolio of initiatives aligned to strategic imperatives; the approach to shaping and resourcing projects is more realistic; and there is simply more use of the tools and techniques of project management. However, many of the old problems and challenges remain—for example, leadership of the project, getting and keeping skilled project managers, and engaging stakeholders and managing their pursuit of their interests.

Our research indicates that the use of projects is widespread throughout the industry, and organisations of all types and sizes have established their own approaches to project management as part of their organisational strategy, with some impressive outcomes to show for their efforts. The organisations represented in our study reported running from three to fifty major projects in a year. Their projects included building and IT (with capital projects having the highest budgets), developing new services and new service delivery models, leading major national initiatives to improve aspects of the service delivery system, quality improvement initiatives, and policy development and research projects. Organisational change was a constant underlying theme.

Participants were positive about projects and their contribution to organisational growth and service improvement and delivery. However, the larger organisations particularly reported difficulty in **controlling** their project agenda for several reasons. Although there had been improvement since our earlier research, organisations tended to overestimate what was achievable, and some are still struggling with disciplining the initiation and approval processes. In addition, when projects are a response to government initiatives or funding opportunities, delayed approval and decision-making processes may make the projects irrelevant or unfeasible by the time they can be implemented. However, senior leaders and project managers consistently reported that their organisations recognise the importance of project management and have been taking a more proactive role in project initiation (rather than mainly responding to funding opportunities, which was more commonly reported in our previous research). More information from our research results is provided throughout the book.

Project management challenges

General management skills and methods are useful in managing projects, but are not by themselves enough—projects require some approaches, methods and tools different from those used for managing routine operations (Turner & Simister 2000). Project managers aim to ensure that the project's end goal is achieved by planning the project, and then executing and monitoring its progress—while controlling resources effectively—before closing and completing evaluation.

More formally, project management is defined as the application of skills and the use of methods, tools and techniques designed to conduct project activities and to enable organisations to plan, manage and achieve one-off tasks or goals (Meredith & Mantel 2009). Project managers must solve the problems of defining what is needed, planning how to deliver it, managing the required resources in a timely and efficient manner, ensuring successful delivery and bedding down the outcomes. To put it another way, project management is a series of processes to monitor and control the time, cost and quality of projects (Westland 2006).

The need for project management skills is most clearly seen in large and complex projects. For example, the implementation of the case-mix funding model in Australian public hospitals as part of national health reform brought many changes, not only to clinical services and support units but also to administrative systems, financial analysis and reporting and information systems. The use of project management approaches allowed better planning and use of resources and better implementation, as staff worked across departmental boundaries to prepare and cope with the changes. Skilled project management provides a focal point for the work of integrating new functional efforts through a (temporary) organisational structure that supports rather than stifles change (Kerzner 2009).

This is one of many examples of major changes in models of care and policy frameworks since the 1990s. Others include integrated mental health services, family-centred care, multipurpose health centres, shared care programs, transitional care and case management. Project management has been an effective means to design and implement new processes, allocate resources, streamline operations and develop new skills. It also allows new technologies and initiatives to be integrated into the organisations more effectively and efficiently.

Project management is also important in responding to a crisis—for example, in the development and deployment of disaster plans. This is necessarily a multidisciplinary and interagency process that can significantly impact on the wellbeing of the entire community or a whole population.

However, the increasing use of projects means that project management knowledge, skills and abilities are needed by virtually all managers, not only those who specialise in project management. As one participant in our research observed, translating skills into project management doesn't always work:

> I was overseeing someone who was doing a project who just didn't know how to do it. Even though he was a great [professional], he'd worked in the hospital a long time, he just didn't have the skills to put it all together and to know how to consult with people and how to run meetings and how to communicate and how to write a project plan and all of that stuff. I think it's

valuable to have the learning, otherwise it takes a long time and you've got to learn it the hard way.

(Hospital clinical leader)

Project management offers a method for driving development processes and successfully implementing change. Successful project management enables organisations to remain relevant and competitive, and to continuously improve products, services and processes. In fact, many organisations conduct their business through projects, called the management-by-projects approach, in which whole divisions or organisations are structured as groups of projects, with resultant gains in flexibility and speed of response to change (McElroy 1996; Burke 2003). The management-by-projects approach is seen to encourage decentralised management responsibilities, a holistic view of problems, and goal-oriented problem solution processes (Burke 2003). Three of the organisations represented in our research fit this description.

The translation of management tools and techniques from industry generally to the health sector is often difficult, requiring major alterations to suit the sector. Sometimes the promised benefits are not realised. Project management is just such an adopted method, and much of the literature does not adequately address the problems that arise in an industry so dominated by skilled professional labour, and so intimately linked to the processes and complexities of government and public policy. This raises two questions: What problems are encountered in the sector? And are the methods of project management robust enough for application in the sector?

Like any tool, project management can be well or badly suited to its chosen use, and can be well or badly used. Properly used, it has the potential to enhance the organisation's ability to innovate and grow, bring discipline to the processes of change, and enable organisations to focus more strongly on their purpose and the outcomes they need to achieve. In our attempt to provide insights into effective use of projects, we believe it is important to proceed from an understanding of the current realities of project management practice in the industry. So we turned first to an analysis of the typical problems encountered in project management in health and community services, based on our research. We found several challenges, which organisations need to meet in order to maximise their gains from the projects they conduct, described in Table 1.1.

Table 1.1 Project management challenges in the health and community services sector

Challenges	Details
The agenda: strategy or opportunism	Ideally, projects contribute to the achievement of organisational strategic directions. However, projects in health and community services are often the result of responses to changes in government policy and initiatives, and to funding opportunities. Although we have seen improvements in the last ten years in how projects are initiated as a result of 'real needs from the organisation', this balance is still hard to keep. Organisations are facing the challenges of getting real benefits out of all the projects they have committed to.
Contested ground: 'You can't change that!'	Projects have been widely used to achieve change. However, change is difficult in the complex and politicised environment of health and community services, with multiple empowered stakeholders and the conditions for effective resistance. Various parts of the organisation may have very different goals, and operate under different and conflicting incentives. Projects flounder and sometimes fail because they are trying to achieve things that are at odds with the team or organisational culture, or which require unwelcome change in work practices, power relationships or ways of working together; or simply because they are are too big to 'chew'.
Hope is not a method	People working in health and community services are accustomed to living with complex goals that outstrip the ability of their organisations to deliver, and with the resultant unmet expectations of the community. Staff are often strongly motivated by altruism, pride and a desire to achieve the best possible outcomes for their clients, their organisations and themselves, and this may lead to a mismatch between the small size of their resources and their much larger goals. Sometimes, projects are designed to convince policy-makers and other key players to pursue a social policy goal by demonstrating how it can work in practice. This strategy can succeed, but issues like 'on time and on budget' are hardly relevant when 'specifications' are a moving target, or have many shapes in the eyes of several different stakeholders.
Making it happen: skills, leadership and teamwork	The leadership challenge in project management occurs at two levels: the authorising level and within the project team. Leadership is a disseminated role in health and community services, which is both a strength and weakness for project

	management. Because project managers must often acquire access to or temporary control of resources that are the responsibility of functional managers and departments, there can be a problem in determining who has the authority to make decisions about issues on which the project's success depends. There is also a problem with conflicting loyalties among those staff who are temporarily seconded to a project—commitment to the project and the project team on the one hand, and to their ongoing functional group on the other. Good project outcomes depend on good project management, and on organisations successfully managing these potential conflicts.
Knowing how: tools, techniques and methods	Although the use of project management methods and tools is important to project success, they are usually more available to large and relatively well-resourced organisations. Because these tools were designed and tested in general industry, they often give inadequate attention to the complexities of multiple stakeholders, multiple agendas and the politics of change that so often underlie project failure in the health and community services sector. Furthermore, the tools themselves may be too rigid to use when most projects in the sector require a high level of flexibility.
Sustainability: did we get there?	The goal of testing the new ideas through successful completion of projects is to implement ongoing programs or services. The project benefits can prove difficult to sustain if little thought has been given to how results might be integrated, or what level of resources and support will be needed to sustain them. Another challenge is how to develop and sustain the organisation's project capacity—keeping their good project managers, and embedding the skills of project management as part of their organisational knowledge.

Is it the sector or is it the method?

In Table 1.1, we outline six challenges that the sector needs to address to get the maximum value from its use of the project approach. An alternative explanation needs to be considered. Are these issues indicators of weaknesses in the method rather than of problems in the sector?

In a sense, projects are simply segments of the ongoing, complicated and sometimes messy business of the organisation in which they sit, with an artificial line drawn around them and some special rules and resources applied. The theoretical model of the project gives it a clear, uncontested goal, a set of technical requirements that must be fulfilled to meet the goal, and a set of methods and tools for doing so. The results are then handed back to grateful operating units, which use them to move forward to a brighter, more effective and more competitive future.

However, it is sometimes argued that the growing use of projects is causing new problems. Managers are often uncomfortable with an approach that requires them to make an upfront commitment to a concrete goal and detailed plan, partly because to do so may reduce their own discretion or power (Partington 1996). Public sector organisations work with complex goals and contested structures, policies and methods. Internal projects must deal with stakeholders who are in effect both the subjects and the objects of change—that is, the change makers and the changed. Thus, the project team may need to change the roles, mindsets or privileges of the very people who must endorse the project's goals and outcomes. In addition, projects may bring their own bureaucracy and, paradoxically, are resistant to change in the project itself while advocating the use of projects to pursue organisational change. Finally, if the methods of project management are not built on an adequate research and theory base, their claims to universal application cannot be justified. A number of our study participants reinforced the importance of having well-tested standardised tools and processes to guide project development and implementation:

> We need a prioritisation process that is standardised, has set criteria and the projects run according to what we actually do. Projects have to demonstrate that they are going to add value to patient access, safety, all the usual things—cost effectiveness, productivity, all those sorts of things, evidence-based practice.
>
> *(Senior hospital manager)*

This book is our answer to the question that started this section: is the method sufficiently robust to serve the needs of the health and community services sector? And the answer is 'yes, for the right purposes and with modifications'. The rest of this book outlines how and why.

Project success and critical success factors

The literature has identified the importance of certain **critical success factors** (CSF) in achieving the project's desired outcomes, on the basis of studies of project success since the 1960s. However, it is also recognised that project success can be defined rather differently in different project contexts and from different perspectives (Belout & Gauvreau 2004).

Early studies of project management tended to focus on reasons for project failure rather than project success. Basically, if a project did not meet one of the '3Ds'—if it was not on time, within budget and meeting the aims of the client—it was a failure (Belassi & Tukel 1996). In reality, the picture is much more complex—many projects go over time and budget but are still judged to be successful by participants for a variety of other reasons.

Table 1.2 gives examples of how project success may be defined from three important perspectives: those of project **sponsors** (this may

Table 1.2 Defining project success from different perspectives

Project sponsor (may be senior management of the organisation)	• Have the expected benefits been achieved? • Have the potential long-term gains been maximised? • Have we funded the right people to do the job, leading to the best return for the financial investment? • Have we funded the right projects to justify the financial investment? • Has the project contributed to achieving organisational objectives (from senior management's perspective)?
Project manager	• Has the project been completed on schedule? • Has the project been completed within budget? • Have all activities been completed and all 'outputs' delivered as planned? • Have changes been managed according to sponsors' expectations along the way? • Have any detrimental effects or risks been minimised? • Has the project team stayed motivated and focused? • Have the key stakeholders been well managed?
Consumer	• Have we received the best services/products possible? • Have the benefits from the services been maximised? • Are the benefits sustainable? • Is this the best way to meet my needs and address my concerns? • Are the overall outcomes of the project satisfactory?

Sources: Pinto and Slevin (1988); Belout and Gauvreau (2004); Shanhar et al. (2005); Shenhar and Dvir (2007); Ika (2009); Assudani and Kloppenborg (2010)

include senior management of the organisation), project managers and consumers.

In addition, the environmental context needs to be considered. Researchers have found that projects often have unexpected side-effects, 70 per cent of which could be attributed to lack of awareness of the environment (White & Fortune 2002). These authors suggest that in many of the methods used, 'insufficient account was taken of project boundaries and environments' (White & Fortune 2002: 5). Some of the side-effects were beneficial to the organisation—for example, an increase in business, sales or opportunities, or gaining new knowledge and understanding. However, the undesirable effects were wide ranging and included organisational conflicts and problems with staff, clients, contractors and/or suppliers, as well as technical limitations. Some organisations reported that the project resulted in greater organisational complexity (Meredith & Mantel 2009). An example in health and community services is that health promotion projects may lead to increases in demand for care.

It is important for staff involved in projects to understand that, in reality, even successful projects may not lead to further actions or result in new services or program development—as one senior health manager noted: 'projects don't always result in action and I think people get confused by that'. Sometimes, a project may prove the ideas proposed will not work or will not produce the intended benefits. Therefore, no set rules can be used to quantify project success, and it cannot be judged without reference to the views of those who are involved and affected.

Determinants of success

We conducted a **systematic literature review** of recent studies of project success (published between 2004 and 2012). The results, although mostly from studies in other sectors, were similar to those reported by participants in our research. A number of factors that contribute to project failure have been identified in research, such as poor time and budget management; a lack of support from key stakeholders; an uncoordinated approach within the project or the organisation; too many scope changes during the project; and unrealistic expectations leading to the establishment of unachievable project goals (Hartley 2009).

The most significant study on CSFs (Pinto & Slevin 1988) identified ten factors that determine success regardless of project type. These factors have been further tested and mainly reinforced by a number of subsequent studies (Fortune & White 2006; Andersen et al. 2006; Mishra et al. 2011). The ten critical factors are:

- project mission (clear goals and direction)
- top management support
- project planning
- client consultation (engagement of stakeholders)
- people management
- technical tasks (having the needed technology and expertise)
- client acceptance (**sign-off**)
- monitoring and feedback
- communication
- trouble-shooting.

Of all the factors, project quality (including clear vision and goals), strong leadership and effective communications have been consistently highlighted (for example, Chen 2011, Rosacker et al. 2010; Assudani & Kloppenborg 2010). The major difference between our results and the published studies is the strong focus on the system and policy influences on projects by our participants, which is not prominent in the published studies. This probably reflects the characteristics of the health and community services sector, and its closeness to policy and politics.

Model for success

Long lists of critical success factors can be daunting, and may include elements that tend to be related ('top management support', for example, is usually correlated with having good access to technology and skills). To ensure the usefulness of the analysis of CSFs in practice, we must organise the wealth of possible elements into categories that make sense and also clarify the cause and effect relationships between them. Drawing on the published research, our research on current project management practice in the sector, and our own experience, we have developed a model that incorporates the main insights and strategies needed by organisations and project managers to ensure that they use project management methods well and get value from their projects. The model is adapted from important work by Belassi and Tukel (1996), which attempts to categorise the success factors meaningfully, and distinguish between underlying organisational and environmental factors and direct project variables.

The success model can be used for checking that key issues have been addressed in project planning and design, as well as for understanding the implications of emerging problems and developing remedial action. It can also be useful for evaluation of project success and failure, and for analysing how the organisation's overall project capacity and success rate might be improved. Finally, it could be used by those who design funding programs and submission guidelines for projects—as a check to ensure that the requirements and criteria they include are consistent with funding successful projects. It is important to note that the factors included in the model may affect projects differently at different **stages** of the project life cycle.

The success factor model (see Figure 1.3) has two major components. The 'project factors' on the right-hand side represent the direct

Figure 1.3 Model for success factors

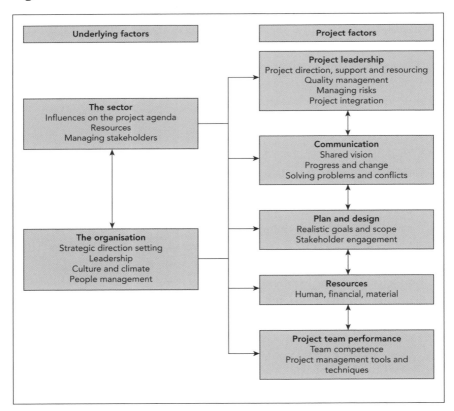

Source: Adapted from Belassi and Tukel (1996)

determinants, or the reality of what happens with projects—what you can see happening on the ground. These features, while critical to project success in their own right, are at least partly outcomes of the interplay of the 'underlying factors' on the left-hand side. The underlying factors are the conditions or enablers that together influence the project experience and outcomes, and they are grouped in two categories or levels—factors in the sector, and factors in the organisation.

Project factors

This model proposes five main categories of direct determinants of project success.

Project leadership: Strong leadership was highlighted not only in the literature but also by our study participants. It is critical that the project sponsor and manager have a good understanding of the way the organisation actually works and the dynamics of its external and internal environment (including the team). Strong project leadership will ensure a project is well founded, aligned with organisational strategic direction, and has clear goals and measurable objectives. Strong leadership is also about building successful relationships, not only with project staff but also with project stakeholders. Strong leadership is not about telling people what to do or what not to do; rather, it is about motivating people to do their job better and allowing the project team to manage their work locally without too much interference.

Communication: Effective communication is critical, and is not limited to the project team but also includes senior management and all significant stakeholders. In an interesting study of the impact of success factors, Andersen and colleagues (2006) found that 'rich project communications' was a surprisingly significant factor—more important, for example, than tight project organisation and control (Andersen et al. 2006: 142–3). As one senior manager put it:

> You've really got to keep communicating with people so they understand what it is you're doing and why you're doing it, so really involving people, listening to them, understanding what their issues are.
>
> *(Hospital clinical leader)*

Plan and design: A good project plan starts with setting clear, achievable goals and objectives. The fundamental vision for a project should remain clear and relatively stable throughout the project life span (Roberts 2011), and be supported with a feasible plan and design. In a longitudinal study of 121 capital projects, Chen (2011) found that the **effectiveness** of the project initiation and planning phases had a significant impact on project success. Without a clear vision and plan, project deliverables/benefits cannot be clearly defined (and later measured), and the project is unlikely to meet expectations or achieve the benefits expected by stakeholders.

Resources: This category includes having skilled people, enough money and the right technology and material resources. Having the right tools, methods, standards and processes is also important, as expressed by a consulting manager: 'Protocols . . . had to be developed and everyone on the team had to know what they were and know how to deal with it . . .'

Project team performance: The final direct success factor is the capacity of the project team to deliver. Does the project team work well? Is it able to manage the change required by the project and to communicate effectively with stakeholders? Is the project team able to use the right project management tools and techniques to maximise the project performance and benefits? As one senior manager put it: 'some of it is just perseverance and tenacity and managing up'.

Underlying factors

The direct factors are not the whole story. Some organisations are more able to get good results from all their projects, and some environmental influences affect all organisations. A suitable internal environment and structure will not only nurture the project to maturity, but also allow the project to progress in a timely way.

We have divided the underlying factors into two major areas.

The sector: This is the environmental context in which organisations, and thus their projects, sit. We have identified three major factors here: the first is the role of government and key stakeholders in influencing the project agenda; the second is having resources available to allow good ideas to be turned into projects; and the third is the critical task of managing the complex relationships with stakeholders that characterise the sector.

The organisation: Some characteristics of organisations are linked to their capacity for project success, including having a strong shared sense of organisational strategy, organisational leadership, a positive culture and supportive climate, and good people-management practices.

The underlying factors that influence success or failure might be less amenable to change, at least for the purposes of a single project, or perhaps not at all. However, the logic of the framework is that attention to these issues—for example, thinking carefully about the 'fit' between the organisation's culture and the project, recognising the industrial issues that the project is likely to encounter and the likely stakeholder concerns—will enable organisations to choose projects, and pursue them, with a maximum chance of success. The industry and organisational factors that enable or constrain project success are discussed in Chapter 2.

Summary

- Projects are a way of achieving a one-off goal, and there is a wealth of methods and tools available to support this work.
- Projects are unique, complex and vary in scope and need to achieve defined goals within clearly defined time, cost and quality constraints.
- Managing a project is not a linear process, but, rather, has a life cycle of four phases: initiation, preparation, implementation and closure.
- The invention of the role of the project manager was a significant breakthrough, enabling organisations to lead and coordinate all the people and resources required for the project to succeed.
- Projects are being used more and more frequently in a world of constant change and increasing complexity, but health and community service organisations are encountering some particular challenges in achieving the anticipated value from their project work and in managing their project portfolios.
- The available critiques of project management have relevance to the sector, and argue for modification of the mainstream methods to suit the needs of the sector (hence this book).
- Project success involves more than achieving the project's intended outcomes within the time and cost allowed—it is also influenced by the interests of internal and external stakeholders and by unintended effects.

- The determinants of project success have been studied in an extensive literature. On the basis of this evidence, we have developed a framework for understanding project success factors and how they relate to one another, with a focus on both the underlying factors in the sector and in organisations, and the direct project management factors such as adequate resources and top management support.
- Most of the existing literature has been designed for engineering, IT and manufacturing industries; this book seeks to fill a gap for the health and community services industry.

Readings and resources

The Australian Institute of Project Management: www.aipm.com.au

Project Management Institute: www.pmi.org

Australian College of Project Management: www.projectmanagement.edu.au/

Association for Project Management: www.apm.org.uk/

Project Management Association of Canada: www.pmac–ampc.ca/

Project Management Institute (PMI) (2008). *A Guide to the Project Management Body of Knowledge* (4th ed). Newtown Square, Pennsylvania: PMI.

Roberts, P. (2011). *Effective project management: identify and manage risk—plan and budget—keep project under control.* London: Kogan Page.

Martin, V. (2002). *Managing projects in health and social care.* New York: Routledge.

Longest, B. B. (2004). *Managing health programs and projects.* San Francisco: Jossey–Bass.

2

The industry, the organisation and project success

In this chapter, we explain aspects of the industry environment that influence project work and the organisational factors that help to determine the chances of project success. We then propose key criteria for choosing and shaping projects that can be adapted and used by leaders and managers to help them make decisions about what projects to do and how to shape them for their own setting (these criteria will also be useful for middle managers seeking to improve their success in getting their projects approved).

The industry: complex, regulated—but still dynamic

Projects are different in different settings, and every industry has characteristics that change the way projects are done. The challenges outlined in Chapter 1 are not unique to health and community services, but they do have particular causes and effects in the sector. For readers without direct experience of working in the sector, the following information explains some important background.

Structural features of the health and community services environment

Government regulation and funding: The industry is highly regulated— and at least partly funded—by government, and so is subject to the vagaries of government policy change and ways of doing business. While this situation creates opportunities for growth, it also restricts strategic choices (particularly for organisations in the public sector) to set their own directions, and requires leaders to find compromises between the demands of government and the needs or priorities of their own organisation. Projects can be part of the problem here (as well as being opportunities), with project portfolios shaped largely by government agendas, regardless of their internal priority.

Dynamic change in policy and practice: The industry is dynamic and most of it is constantly engaged in change and development. This means that there is room to find better ways of working, and it can enable staff to muster great energy and commitment. However, it can also lead to important staff groups pulling in different and sometimes contradictory directions. Leaders are subjected to increasing demands for service development and resource allocation, while budgets and resources are always constrained. Staff get 'change fatigue', and project resources can be spread too thin.

People-rich environment: This is a people-rich industry, with many tertiary-educated staff who are used to exercising professional independence and are organised into powerful professional and trade union groups. Leaders are accustomed to standing on 'contested ground', with some sections of the workforce agitating for change and others (those with something to lose) digging in or refusing to engage. This means that stakeholder engagement is both critical and challenging.

High social values: The critical social role of the industry means that politicians, the media and the community have strong views about services and standards, and this can result in both external pressure for change, and resistance to it. This impacts on the initiatives organisations seek to implement through projects, and on the ways that projects are managed.

In health and community services, there are three main ways that these characteristics of the industry impact directly on the way projects are used (and how well they work). They are the influence of governments on the project agenda; the funding and resourcing of projects; and the challenges of stakeholder management.

Influences on the project agenda: the role of government

Governments and other funders have a major impact on the project portfolios of health and community services. While this is true in both the private and public sectors, it is more acute for government-funded agencies. The impact of government has risen over recent years in many ways, including an increasingly active role as 'purchasers' of particular services (rather than passive subsidisers of provider organisations). This has also brought increased use of project funding as a strategy for encouraging change in practice and models of care, and for enhancing government's ability to monitor and control agencies.

Direct government funding programs for improvement and innovation projects have enabled cash-strapped agencies to invest in updating their services, to bring in new approaches more suited to current needs and technologies, and to enhance their capacity to analyse service data. Eligible organisations develop skills in presenting their priorities in the terms of the funder's policy goals, while also retaining focus on their own goals.

However, our research indicates that governments have changed their approach to stimulating innovation in recent years, and are more likely to rely on centralised development and/or tighter specification of what is to be done. Participants in public hospitals and health services in particular reported increasing use of regulation and performance standards to drive improvement efforts, and less use of direct funding of improvement projects. Leaders in our research (including those in government health departments) reported real constraints in their choice of projects, and increasing requirements to respond to policy and funding changes—for example, tobacco policy, activity-based funding, national emergency access targets, electronic health record implementation and other aspects of continuing national health reform. As noted above, there was also an increased presence of national government-owned organisations that were effectively project-based (that is, structured primarily to deliver a set of projects commissioned by government).

The rapid expansion and major investment in eHealth (health ICT) initiatives is a prime example. As part of the national health reform agenda, the Department of Health and Ageing has invested significantly in two main areas: the National telehealth initiative and the National eHealth record system for Personally Controlled Electronic Health Records (PCeHR). This investment in eHealth has driven a large number of projects, managed by the National E-Health Transition Authority (NeHTA).

The projects cover a broad spectrum of activity including eHealth standards, telehealth, health identifiers, information exchange, health terminologies and software development. They touch every part of the health sector: primary care, community care, health services, health insurers, diagnostic providers, aged care and technology providers. However, given the nature of the work, this round of development needs to be driven centrally, and so the projects tend to be shared nationally with state and territory health authorities and/or be contracted out to major suppliers. The health services are largely recipients rather than drivers of this project agenda, although hospital and health services staff are involved as stakeholders.

Regardless of the methods government use, government policy and funding is and will remain a strong influence on project agendas. This is not in itself a problem—government has a responsibility to determine both policy and the use of tax-payer funds. But health and community service providers have a different set of responsibilities, and different imperatives. They must attend to the capacity of the organisation, to the coordinated delivery of the right services to meet client/patient needs, and to the shaping of a coherent strategy to achieve the agency's purpose, all within usually tight budget constraints. For public sector agencies, their purposes may well have been determined by the funder, but the provider's imperative to make it work remains. In the private sector, many services are funded by government, and government regulation of incentives and standards is an important influence, and sometimes a constraint, on operations and service delivery.

There is thus a real risk that regulation and the availability of funding itself will become too strong a driver of the agency's attention, energy and resources, usurping the role that strategic directions and business strategies should play. Although we have outlined the problems generated by government influence on project decision-making, it must be noted that project funding has also served as a vital source of innovation resources, and that service delivery agencies have often made wise use of the available funding.

Resourcing projects

Participants in our research indicated that competition for project resources within organisations is widespread and important. The most common reasons for project proposals failing to get approval (mentioned by about half of the participants) were financial, and this meant both cost per se and the strength of the **business case**—that is, the potential for the project results to generate a positive financial impact that justified the costs and effort.

For private sector organisations, the direct need to generate a financial return on investment imposes discipline on decisions to authorise projects, while also enabling leaders to support promising projects. In the public sector, cost-saving and cost-neutrality (that is, the criterion that an alternative way of doing things should cost no more than is currently being spent) are important considerations in decision-making. However, there is less capacity to balance costs with enhanced revenue (because revenue is at least partly set by government), which means that it can be very hard to find resources even for important and valuable projects.

This is an enduring feature of the industry, and one that underlies several reasons for project failure, including underbudgeting, inadequate staffing and unrealistic timing.

Managing stakeholders

One of the most difficult challenges in project management in the sector is managing the key stakeholders: the influential people and groups (within and outside the organisation) who are affected by the project, and who usually have different and competing agendas. The risk is that the person with the loudest voice or strongest personality can take a project in an undesirable direction based on a whim or a 'good idea'.

For most projects, internal groups—staff, volunteers, different professions and departments or units—are the main stakeholders. At the industry level there are external stakeholders who might become involved in a project, perhaps through being part of a steering or advisory committee, being a project funder or being part of the project process. Different professional and trade union organisations (and their internal representatives and members) may have their own sectoral interests that are beyond the scope of the project. They can stymie change and derail projects, sometimes deliberately, but sometimes because adherence to their own agendas does not allow them to see any alternatives.

Governments can also be key stakeholders. Government agencies can change their minds and alter their policy directions well into the project life cycle, due to a change in government or a change of key personnel, or because more important priorities come along. Governments are also susceptible to public opinion and political lobbying, and a project that has potential for unpopularity is vulnerable if strong community or political opposition is mobilised against it.

Consumers are another important stakeholder group who can be difficult for professional staff to engage and involve. Staff may question the capacity of consumers to contribute, or feel challenged by a shift in relative roles (from being 'in charge' to engaging as equals). Consumers with a chronic condition might be too ill to participate for very long in a project, other consumers might be transitory and move on to other interests. Consumers can become disillusioned by their experiences in committees or reference groups—perhaps because their expectations are so high that they are never likely to be realised, or because they feel disempowered by the approaches of the professionals involved in the project management process. On the other hand, a lot has been learnt about both goals and effective approaches to involving consumers (see, for example, Hibbard 2003; Consumers Health Forum of Australia 2008).

In many situations the influence of powerful people pulling in different directions leads to 'stakeholder paralysis' where nothing gets done and people become angry and frustrated. Case 2.1 outlines an alternative method for engaging stakeholders in the decision-making process. Maintaining stakeholder engagement throughout the life of the project is also sometimes a challenge. Managing stakeholders is addressed in depth in Chapters 5 and 7.

Case 2.1 Getting beyond stakeholder paralysis

The operating theatres of a major teaching hospital were performing badly on a number of efficiency indicators, and the hospital leadership group was clear that the traditional discipline-based structure was a barrier to improvement. The group discussed setting up a project with the goal of designing a more modern team-based structure. A member of the leadership group had rich experience of change projects becoming bogged down through the creation of steering committees in which all stakeholder interests were represented—and in which representatives set about protecting their sectional interests. He suggested a different approach: that the CEO and a senior clinician (who was identified as not having a structural stake in the question) act as a panel of review, and design the best possible structure for good teamwork. The outcome of their deliberations would be brought back to the group for endorsement and then implemented.

To the CEO's surprise, this suggestion was universally supported, and the two-person team (with project officer support) proceeded to invite submissions and conduct interviews, commission a small literature review and prepare a short report. They recommended structural change to achieve a situation in which all major groups working in the theatres (excluding the surgeons who were defined as 'users' of theatre services) would report to a theatre suite manager and work in multidisciplinary teams.

The CEO's experience was that the process of submissions and interviews enabled the various staff groups to tell some of the real stories and identify the obstacles to improved service; the process also enabled both providers and users to identify the outcomes they sought rather than focusing on the 'ownership' issues. The report was readily accepted, and the momentum for constructive change carried through to successful implementation. The panel's objectivity, and the trust of those directly affected, were identified as key success factors. Trust had been enhanced by a transparent process that was safe for those who participated. In the end, stakeholder interests were heard and incorporated, but the paralysis often encountered in the stakeholder committee structure was avoided.

This is not a classical method of designing a project, but such an approach may be effective when a key decision needs to be made prior to work on implementation. In this case, commitment by all stakeholders in advance made the implementation project easier, quicker and perhaps more effective in the end.

Project capability in organisations

While important environmental and industry factors do have a strong impact on projects, organisational capability is critical (Roberts 2011). The health and community services field is large and diverse, but there are a number of common project success factors at the level of the organisation as a whole: strategic direction setting, leadership, culture (and climate) and approaches to the management of people. Leaders need to recognise these underlying influences, and anticipate and manage their potential positive or negative impact.

Strategic direction setting

Although projects 'stand alone' with their specific goals and objectives, they also need to align with the organisation's strategic goals and be an integrated part of the organisation (Chen 2011). In our research, about half of the participants reported that not being sufficiently well aligned with the organisation's priorities and needs was a common reason for project proposals failing to be approved.

There was overall a stronger sense of control of project agendas than there was in our earlier research, and a greater focus on proper resourcing and project governance. But managers also commented on the temptation to take on too many projects and not give sufficient priority to critical issues. According to a senior hospital manager: 'If you want to succeed, do fewer and dive deep'.

While there was strong reliance on the discipline of the formal processes of development and approval, managers also noted the importance of ensuring that the organisation avoids duplication of effort and has a good strategic understanding of costs and benefits (meaning some projects without a strong financial business case might be approved). There was also a greater emphasis on linking projects to the operational plan or business plan. Several participants spoke about the need to strengthen their decision-making in this regard—for example, by having standardised processes and a set of criteria that project proposals need to meet, including alignment to strategies and business plans:

> The Executive Directors know that if they want to get something onto the project schedule or get it approved because it's of significance they have to bring along a completed project proposal and we would just review it, predominantly against the work plan. Does it help us with [the overarching] purpose? Is it consistent with legislation? Have we got the capacity to do it and what are the resource implications of doing it or not doing it?
>
> *(Government senior manager)*

The impact of the strategic directions and business plans on project success depends on two elements: alignment of projects to the plan, and strength of the plan. Firstly, the success of a project will depend partly on how it aligns with the organisation's strategies for achieving its basic purpose or mission. Secondly, the relative strength of the strategic direction (how strongly and broadly it is supported throughout the organisation) will impact on the ability of the organisation to muster coordinated support for a key project.

The reverse is also true: if the strategic plan is a weak instrument, poorly aligned projects are less likely to be weeded out. It is difficult to use the organisation's strategic plan as a test for the priority of particular funding opportunities if the plan is not strongly understood and valued by the majority of influential people and groups in the organisation. We found this to be a major source of difficulties with managing the project portfolio, and not only in human services. A large study in the US pharmaceutical industry, for example, found that leaders in many of the firms surveyed singled out the organisation's inability to prioritise effectively as a key weakness, caused by 'countervailing organisational special interests' that were able to resist the portfolio-level decisions of senior management (Case 1998: 593).

Most health and community service organisations have a strategic directions document, but in some cases there is not enough commitment or shared understanding throughout the organisation to allow it to drive decision-making from top leadership level down. To look at this another way, the problem is not that there are no strategic directions, but rather that there are several competing and perhaps contradictory ones.

Internal politics is an ongoing reality—the interests of individuals, units and teams within the organisation will not always align with the organisation's broader interests or strategies, and the result is a leadership problem. Neither leaders nor projects can change this reality—part of what is sometimes called the 'shadow side' of organisations (Egan 1994)—but there are strategies for managing it. Strategic plans can be designed to recognise and better align the interests of important internal stakeholders with those of the organisation as a whole. They can also be used in such a way as to channel 'political' activity out of the corridors and into structured priority-setting processes. We return to this difficult question in Chapter 7. Some of the organisations represented in our research were project-based—that is, their strategic direction setting was effectively enacted as a portfolio of projects. This is unusual in the field, but in general there was a shift in the discussion towards stronger control of project agendas.

Leadership at every level

Among all the important organisational elements, support from senior management (or management **buy-in**) is viewed as one of the critical project success factors—not only by our interviewees, but also in the literature (for example, Andersen et al. 2006; Fortune & White 2006; Morteza & Kamyar 2009). One of the major requirements for project success identified by our respondents was effective leadership. Leadership to ensure staff 'own' the project and understand how it fits into the overall direction of the organisation is critical. As several participants said, if you haven't got high-level endorsement and championing, it is very hard to make even a great idea work.

People we interviewed also commented on the difficult leadership task of both generating commitment and simultaneously imposing discipline on project activity, a task that is challenging for all of the reasons outlined earlier in this chapter. This task applies at every level of the organisation, from the board of directors to project team members. For all organisations in our study, projects were an ongoing feature of their work, and they had developed some ongoing capacity to coordinate and support them.

Culture and climate

It has become fashionable to describe organisational cultures according to their relevance for particular goals. Thus management writers and consultants advocate for a 'quality culture', 'innovation culture', 'learning culture' or 'high performance culture', and project management writers are part of this trend (for example, O'Kelly & Maxwell 2001).

Organisation culture is a much-discussed but ill-defined concept, which makes intuitive sense to most people who have worked in organisations but is hard to study and perhaps even harder to manipulate. By culture, we mean the unwritten values and rules that are understood and endorsed by the staff (or important subgroups) and therefore govern 'how things are done around here'.

According to our research, organisations with a culture that supports project success have three key characteristics: they have an ability to handle change; they have the ability to incorporate new knowledge— that is, to learn; and there is a broad awareness among staff of the project method and how it can be used. These characteristics, particularly the first two, are generally also seen as part of those other desired cultures (high performance, quality, and so on), and there is a vast literature on these questions (for example, Leggat & Dwyer 2003; Shore 2008). O'Kelly and Maxwell (2001) argue enthusiastically for the adoption of a project management culture in health care, particularly in relation to the implementation of clinical governance in the UK. For these authors, a project management culture implies an ability to initiate change and get things done in a manageable way through the use of project teams. Organisational leaders cannot change culture at will, but they can understand and encourage those aspects of the culture that support innovation, willingness to learn and the development of shared project capability.

Idealism is an issue for the management of individual projects in health and community services, as well as for the management of project portfolios—and not only in the public sector. Commitment to the 'public good' ethos is seen in committed effort to provide good services regardless of the barriers; in acceptance of ambiguity and complexity; and also in the difficulty experienced by many health and community service organisations in choosing priorities among competing needs or options. When judgements must be made about which worthy project to sacrifice and which to approve, the process of decision-making is often prolonged, emotional, politicised and less strategic than leaders would like to admit.

Perhaps the business culture that produced modern project management is more pragmatic, with more concrete goals and more direct methods of pursuing them, than is the health and community services culture. It is hard to imagine the slogan 'faster, better, cheaper', with its implication of uncomplicated acceptance of a clear and concrete goal, becoming a rallying cry in human services. Ideals like 'quality, access, equity' are both more familiar, and more abstract and complex.

The concept of team or organisational climate is perhaps more directly amenable to leadership attention. If culture is defined as 'how we do things around here', climate is 'how it feels to work here'. Climate can be changed profoundly by good leadership. There are six main elements that taken together constitute the settings for high performance (see the list below). There is good evidence (for example, Edmondson 1999) that a team climate in which the leader enables staff to feel safe in questioning accepted ways of doing things creates the conditions for success in innovation. This is an important insight for leaders who seek to enhance the chances of project success.

Team climate is set according to how staff perceive their working environment in relation to these six elements (HRM Advice 2008):

- Flexibility—are staff free to innovate?
- Responsibility—how free are staff to work without asking for permission and guidance from the manager?
- Standards—are goals high but attainable?
- Rewards—is good work recognised, through direct feedback and/or tangible rewards?
- Clarity—do staff know what is expected from them and how that relates to the organisational goals?
- Team commitment—do staff know they belong to a winning team or organisation and that goals are shared?

While team commitment is positive, the related idealism that is part of health and community services culture can be a source of resistance to change. The 'missionary organisation' (Mintzberg 1991) is one that pursues values-based goals (like relieving suffering or reducing inequality) and attracts staff who are personally driven by those goals. Their commitment, however, may lead them to resist what they perceive as incorrect interpretations of the mission. When this tendency is linked to self-interest (for example, a proposed change to a model of service that will require change in patterns of work) it can be a powerful force. Any attempt to change the way that things are done can be seen as an attack on the fundamental values and philosophies of the organisation, and as a threat to service quality and commitment to consumers. We return to this point in Chapter 7 when we explore the management of change.

We have found in our teaching, as well as in the interviews for this book, that health and community services staff can have difficulty accepting some of the basic features of the project method: the limited goals, the emphasis on concrete 'deliverables', and the importance of questions like 'will it be finished by the end of next month?'.

Experience in the organisations we surveyed tends to support this conclusion. The common experience of failure (or disappointing results) in change and innovation projects can often be seen to proceed from the failure to free the project itself from the entrenched interests that can be predicted to resist change. The idea of enhancing culture and climate may seem like a forlorn hope to embattled project managers and organisation leaders. Culture change may be difficult and slow, but attention to culture is useful for two reasons. Firstly, even difficult and slow changes have to begin somewhere, and projects can make a significant contribution to culture change. Secondly, the savvy project manager needs to see clearly, and work with and around, the cultural barriers they can't change.

People management and project skills

Project capacity can also be built through attention to the people side of organisations in two specific ways: in finding and keeping good project managers; and in embedding the skills of project management as part of the organisation's knowledge.

Almost all the project management literature and all the participants in our research spoke about the importance of having the right staff. This will not be achieved by placing people in project manager roles because they have a good idea and want to be the one to implement it; or because they are good at something else; or because you have nothing else for them to do and need to find them a job. These practices may be more common in the sector than in industry generally (Rosacker et al. 2010). To avoid these problems, some organisations 'buy in' project managers from outside, either as consultants or as temporary employees. This can work well but is not always a satisfactory solution—consultants can be expensive, they might not fit in with organisational culture easily, and they might not be very good despite their glowing references and marketing. The same applies to temporary project managers—by the time you find out that they haven't really got the skills you thought they had, you are halfway through the project.

It may be more strategic to identify and keep good project managers within the organisation. Skills that are seen as valuable for project management such as communication, negotiation, facilitation, change and conflict management are valuable for all managers. The temporary nature of projects, and particularly the timing of project funding, also means that organisations need to focus on embedding the learning and skills gained through their projects, and on retaining corporate knowledge. This can be difficult if project managers are contract staff and their contracts come to an end, when the learning and corporate memory will depart with them unless an emphasis is placed on adequate handover and documentation.

Projects in government departments

Government looms large in project management in the public sector, with central departments being involved at several levels. Their programs generate and direct a lot of the project activity in service delivery agencies. They also conduct or commission a large number of projects as part of their own responsibilities, and they too experience difficulties managing their project portfolios. Government is an area where the ideal of fixed goals and timelines is particularly hard to achieve.

Much of the work of staff in government departments can be defined as projects. The development of policies and standards, and the tendering of programs and services, are common examples. The processes of project definition and project approval have a political as well as a bureaucratic component, and the birth of projects may be particularly complicated in sensitive and newly emerging policy areas. Projects emerge and take shape from the interplay of political decision-making; interpretations at the governance level of the department; and less-elevated operational processes.

A consultant we interviewed for the first edition of this book stated this strongly—'government manages by projects'—and identified three main reasons for the extensive use of external consultants. Firstly, at state level, periodic reductions in the size of the public sector workforce and the resultant loss of 'good people' have made it harder for departments to contribute to policy development. Executives must often choose between 'treading water' (and thereby making little progress on major issues) or using outsourced intellectual capability. Secondly, external consultants are used for 'leapfrogging quick change', especially in politically sensitive areas where major policy jigsaws need to be managed. Thirdly, external players are seen as being more objective, while also bringing the benefit of the transfer of skills to departmental staff.

In the rest of this book we turn to the models and methods of project management that are the immediate influences on project success, and which we have argued are supported or constrained by the industry and organisational factors outlined above. But first, we want to apply the industry and organisational analysis to the question of project strategy: the decisions organisations make about what project opportunities to pursue, and how they manage their overall project effort. In the rest of this chapter, we present some criteria for use in selecting and approving projects—the organisation's 'project portfolio' is the sum of these choices.

The project or the plan

The rational planning approach to developing a project portfolio is embodied in *A Guide to the Project Management Body of Knowledge* (PMI 2008) and reflected in many textbooks (for example, Haynes 1994; Dobson 1996; Rosenau 1998; Verzuh 2011). The strategic plan is the first step; followed by the development of services, or programs of activity, to implement the plan; and then the commissioning of projects to develop, enable, support or modify the activities. Thus programs are related to organisation strategy, and ongoing program management (for example, managing a fundraising program) is supported by project management (for example, staging a breast cancer ball).

The rational approach was reflected in the way some of our informants described their practice. Several had instituted organised methods for developing project proposals, designing criteria for their approval, ranking proposals against one another, selecting those to be approved (either for internal funding or to be included in bids for external funding), and resourcing and coordinating the resultant activities.

In larger organisations, these processes were generally applied to sets of potential projects that were seen to be truly competing with one another for endorsement and resources within a division or program (such as quality improvement, or buying new equipment)—rather than at the level of the organisation as a whole. Some smaller organisations had a single system for ranking and approving projects, ensuring coherence and manageability through a comprehensive annual priority-setting process. Most of the managers we interviewed had experienced growing acceptance of the discipline of sticking to the strategic plan, often as a result of the pain of failing to do so:

> Some projects seem to be a waste of money and prevent other initiatives getting done. Sometimes [government] priorities take precedence or are competing with internal priorities.
>
> *(Hospital project director)*

The rational planning method has many attractions, but often cannot be achieved. Participants in our research nominated several reasons why the strategic plan might not help at the time the decisions about individual projects have to be made. These reasons include restructuring that has left the status of the strategic plan unclear, or up for review; the appointment of a new CEO and leadership team; or the fact that the strategic plan only deals with service delivery issues and is insufficient as a guide to prioritising project decisions in support areas.

In spite of these limitations, our research and the literature indicate that it is useful to cling to the plan as much as possible and to develop open, predictable, rational methods for prioritising projects. Taking this basic proposition as a starting point, the next task is to develop criteria and methods for selecting the project portfolio.

Criteria for ranking and selecting the project portfolio

The goal of selection of projects has been described as the search for 'a paddock of thoroughbreds' (Case 1998)—that is, each project should be well designed and capable of delivering the desired results. The criteria actually used for adopting projects into a portfolio will be unique to each organisation, and probably to the program or business area, and will change over time. Different criteria will get different weightings, sometimes overtly, sometimes covertly. Alignment with the organisation's strategic intent is often espoused as the major criterion, but decisions can always be influenced by other agendas, or simply by a rush of enthusiasm. Having explicit criteria, and a rigorous process for applying them, is a safeguard against the influence of organisational politics or an excess of zeal, but not a guarantee. On the other hand, not having explicit criteria is an almost guaranteed method of ensuring that many of the wrong horses get into the paddock. The ideas presented below are based on the project success model developed in Chapter 1, and are expressed as generic templates or principles that might be used in designing criteria.

Will this project help to achieve our strategic goals, directly or indirectly? We have said that this is really the starting point, but for many health and community service organisations the goals are so broad that even moderately skilled enthusiasts can make a case for almost anything under this criterion. Goal-setting theory tells us that specific goals are more motivating than vague general ones (Latham & Locke 1979), and in this case specific strategic goals are more useful as criteria. If the strategic directions statement or business plan is not specific enough, it can be modified into a statement of strategic goals for projects in the organisation, borrowing legitimacy from the main statement while making it more readily useful for project portfolio management.

There might be times when organisations decide to take on projects that do not fit clearly within their strategic directions and there might be good reasons for doing so. For example, you might want to explore a particular issue to see if it is something you should take up or in order to develop a relationship with a particular group or funding body. The strategic goals of the funders are also important, and sometimes it is worth being flexible on the alignment question in order to participate in important initiatives of governments and other funders. If this is the case, it is vital to be clear about why you are doing it and what you will do if it does or does not work out.

Does it fit with our culture and values, or what we want them to be—really? We have emphasised the importance of aligning the project portfolio with the organisation's strategic directions, but we have also noted the difficulties human service organisations experience in moving in a coordinated way. Culture clash is a powerful source of some of these difficulties: 'Culture eats strategy for lunch' (attributed to Edgar Schein). We are not suggesting that projects that challenge the prevailing culture should be avoided. Rather, we are saying that the barriers must be identified and a method for dealing with them factored into the project plan—either through clever avoidance or through effective change management strategies.

Another way of thinking about this is to consider the fact that many projects are focused on achieving improvement through changing the way operational processes work. Such projects occupy the 'white spaces in the organisation chart' (Rummler & Brache 1995); that is, they focus on processes in which typically several teams or departments are involved—and no-one is in charge. This is also the area where much of the feral culture of the organisation is created.

Our second criterion suggests that it is worthwhile to check the project fit with the culture and values in two ways. Firstly, does the project, its goals and methods, sit well with the values we aspire to? And, secondly, will this project encounter strong resistance because it cuts across some of the strongly held imperatives of the 'shadow side' of the organisation, the values or practices we may wish were different (noting that sometimes shadow-side values and practices are positive)?

If the answer to the second question is 'yes', then decisions must be made as to whether the project offers a good opportunity to challenge these values and practices, and how this might be done. The other option is to look for ways of avoiding the point where the clash of values occurs. It may be, however, that the culture problem is so strong that the project is doomed to failure and should not be taken on.

Is this a project or an elephant? We have discussed the problem of mistaking hope for a workable method—having a good idea, or a worthy aspiration, does not necessarily translate into a feasible project. Projects need both a goal and a practical method—they need to be clearly defined, concrete and achievable within a timeframe that can be reasonably estimated. Without a method, you may have a pressing problem or a great opportunity, but you will not have a project. The means of solving the given problem, or taking advantage of the opportunity, need to be clearly identified and available.

Is there a leader for this project—a sponsor who will make sure it delivers? Lack of leadership was seen as a problem by several of our informants, at two levels. The first is the level of the project team (see Chapter 7), but here we are focusing on the second— someone in a leadership position who is prepared to sponsor or champion this project, to be the person who will provide influence and access to needed resources when the team requires it. 'Top management support' is often cited in the project management literature as a make-or-break factor (for example, White & Fortune 2002), and our research supports this. But the level and type of support that is needed will vary widely depending on the project and the organisation's structure and style.

Does this project require partners and, if so, is this feasible? Failure to recognise the external implications of projects is a common problem reported in the literature, including White and Fortune's large study (2002). Our informants spoke often of the need for effective partnerships to achieve many of the service development projects they had embarked upon.

The challenge is to recognise the need for partnerships in the early stages and to manage them well. Organisations that are more engaged with their environments and their communities, and which have established more robust relationships, are better placed both to see the implications and to move quickly to respond to them.

Do we have, or can we readily get, the skills to succeed with this project? Again, we are referring not only to project management skills, but also to the core competencies of the organisation—are we innovators or implementers? Do we have the basic technological know-how to support this project and its results? Are we in a position to work well with the intended client group, and with the key funders and regulators?

This criterion can also be used for consideration of the human resource questions—will this project provide good opportunities for the development of project skills and for career development?

Can we handle the resource requirements in a timely manner? This question is not simply about accurate estimation and securing the direct funding requirements of the project—these issues will be addressed in Chapters 5 and 6. The question here is about the capability of the organisation to mobilise the skills, staffing and management attention required to support effective project management.

If it succeeds, are the results sustainable? This was an important problem for most of the organisations we studied, and one that is often deferred. 'We won't know 'til we get there' may often be true. And sometimes you need to demonstrate a successful approach in order to generate the conditions for acceptance and resourcing. But organisations should include consideration of this kind of project risk in their planning and decision-making.

Will this project contribute to our organisational learning and competence? Related to the theme of sustainability is the question of the potential for projects to contribute to the development of the organisation, its core competencies and organisational learning. We argue that this learning and development potential should rank strongly as a criterion when the project portfolio is being compiled.

The 'which projects should we do?' checklist summarises our analysis of project portfolio selection. It is necessarily generic—we suggest that individual organisations could refine the list to focus it more strongly on their unique considerations.

Checklist: which projects should we do?

- Will this project help to achieve our strategic goals, directly or indirectly?
- Does it fit with our culture and values, or what we want them to be—really?
- Is it a project or an elephant?
- Is there a leader for this project—a sponsor who will make sure it delivers?
- Does this project require partners and, if so, is this feasible?
- Do we have, or can we readily get, the skills to succeed with this project?
- Can we handle the resource requirements in a timely manner?
- If it succeeds, are the results sustainable?
- Will this project contribute to our organisational learning and competence?

Summary

- The health and community services sector is strongly regulated, but also dynamic and constantly changing.
- There are three key influences that enable or constrain project success across the sector:
  - tension between strategy (sticking to the plan) and opportunism (brought on by enthusiasms or by the availability of funding)
  - the tendency to overestimate what can be achieved and underestimate time and resources
  - the influence of multiple empowered stakeholder groups.
- Government departments are deeply involved in project work, and experience a clash between the project management approach and the complexities and vagaries of government policy and bureaucracy.

- Government offers significant funding for projects, but increasingly is also controlling and managing the project agenda centrally.
- There are four key factors that underlie the capability of organisations to succeed in project management: strategic direction, leadership, supportive culture and climate, and good people management (including building and maintaining project skills).
- Based on evidence about project success factors, criteria for senior managers to use in choosing which projects to support can be specified. They can also be used by middle managers as a guide to pitching their project proposals.

Readings and resources

On organisational culture and climate:

Unwritten Ground Rules: www.ugrs.net/index_newlook.html

HRM advice: hrmadvice.com/hrmadvice/hr-strategy/the-organizational-climate.html

On engaging consumers:

Health Issues Centre Resource Library: www.healthissuescentre.org.au/subjects/list-library-subject.chtml?subject=24

On investment in eHealth:

National E-Health Transition Authority: www.nehta.gov.au

3

Understanding project management

> Project management careers
> Project management seminars, courses and professional
> development
> **Summary**

Many of the people involved in new developments and innovation in health and community services, ourselves included, have learnt by doing. That is, we have taken a rational approach to the planning and implementation of something new and used our managerial skills to ensure that it gets done. However, not all staff have had managerial training or experience, and we found the practice of expecting competent professional staff to be able to 'just do' project management to be a common problem in the sector:

> Everybody was doing it, no consistent methodology, no systematic reporting . . . no systematic risk management and really no way of knowing whether things were beginning, ending, proceeding, and then sometimes you'd actually find a project would then kind of morph into an ongoing thing.
>
> *(Government senior manager)*

We also found that these activities are still sometimes not identified or managed as projects, although this problem seems to be less common than it was in our earlier research. In this chapter we explain the foundations of project management as a method, and outline the emergence of careers in project management in the sector.

The terminology of project management

In the project management literature there are lots of acronyms—for example, PERT (**program evaluation and review technique**) and WBS (**work breakdown structure**)—and technical terms such as **Gantt chart**, '**close-out**', '**go-live**', 'project scope' and 'deliverables'. It seems that project management has a language all of its own. The use of project terminology can be confusing—it is not necessarily consistent, and sometimes the terms are simply alternative labels for the activities that managers do as part of their daily work: setting goals and targets, deciding on strategy, working out tasks and responsibilities and evaluating. However, the terms are helpful, and are widely used by project managers and in project management literature. The Glossary at the beginning of the book defines some common project management terms.

The project life cycle

The project life cycle—initiate, plan, implement and close—is a model that explains the normal progression of projects to completion (Kloppenborg 2009). Its use assists project teams to plan and monitor progress (see Figure 1.2). But it is not necessarily a simple linear process. Instead, there may be many cycles of planning, implementation, evaluation and variation, which in turn are the subject of reflection. Thus the project life cycle is often used to refocus and reframe activities, and project management then includes a reflective learning process.

The first phase of the cycle, *initiate*, involves the identification of a problem or opportunity and some initial concept development and scoping. This is the 'good idea' stage. It is common for organisations to have a process for documenting and sifting these good ideas before any more detailed work is done. Those that pass this test enter the second phase, *plan*. This involves exploration and analysis focused initially on clarifying the goals; and then on defining the scope (how big is it?); and finally on preparing a plan for how and when and by whom the project will be done, what resources are required and how success will be judged. The results of this stage are generally captured in a project plan, which may go through more than one version with checking and adjustments as details are added.

The third phase, which commences when the project plan is approved, is to *implement*. This is where the work happens, and all involved need to work together to get the tasks of the project completed. Managing this phase requires that the project's progress is tracked and corrected if needed, and that the tendency to drift into extra work or to change the original aims is also managed (sometimes through accepting change, sometimes by sticking to the plan). Implementation also includes ensuring that the costs don't blow out, that the needed 'deliverables' are in fact produced, and that the needed data and information are recorded.

The fourth phase is *close*, when the process of handover, or transitioning from the project to the new method or state, is completed.

In this phase, final reports are submitted; all project documentation is completed and handed over; an evaluation of the project's success and the learnings is completed; and final communications and celebrations are held and thanks expressed.

Although these phases are presented sequentially, during the actual project several of the phases may occur concurrently or repeatedly (in projects with more than one stage, or as plans need to change). The use of repeated cycles of the project management method is diagrammatically represented in Figure 3.1.

Figure 3.1 The iterative nature of the project life cycle

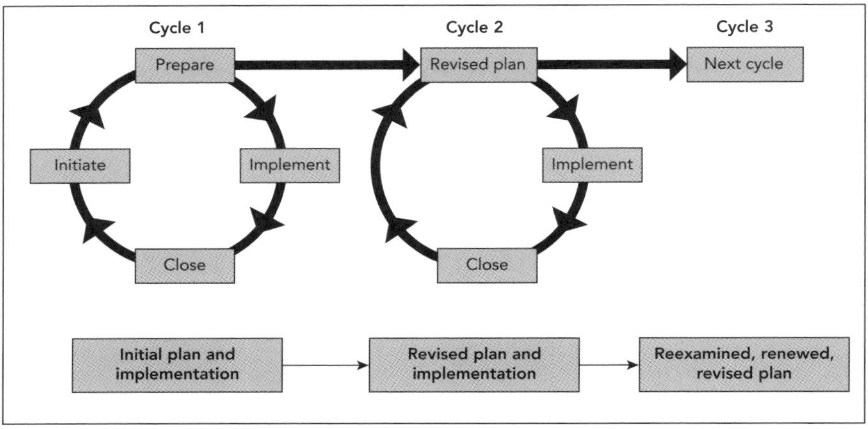

Source: Adapted from Martini (2006)

Multistage projects

As well as having a life cycle, projects may be divided into more than one stage, to make a large or complex project more manageable, and sometimes because each stage has associated outputs or 'deliverables' (that is, tangible, verifiable work products) (PMI 2008). For example, a project that aims to acquire and implement a new information system for registering clients of a mental health service will have at least one **'go/no go'** decision point—that is, the time at which the organisation decides whether to accept the chosen system. Work before and after that point can be seen as two cycles (initiate, plan, implement and close) within the larger project or, in other words, as two separate stages. Other stages might also be required—for example, following technical installation and testing it may be useful to manage the remaining work as a separate stage of the project. There may be significant aspects of the commissioning process that require new planning, execution and closure (such as the conduct of staff training, the transfer of existing data and 'go-live' commissioning) which were unable to be planned before the system was tested.

As can be seen from this example, defining project stages and their outputs enables progressive decisions to be made about whether or not to move on to the next stage. This would normally take the form of a requirement for 'sign-off' (formal acceptance by the client or sponsor of the project) before the next stage could proceed. Many projects do not continue after the completion of a stage for a variety of reasons—perhaps they were found not to be feasible, or were not able to be completed within acceptable timeframes, or were simply not important enough to the organisation.

The number of stages and the activities or deliverables in each stage depend entirely on the project and the industry within which it is being carried out.

Examples of project life cycles

A generic statement of the project life cycle and two examples are provided in Table 3.1.

All projects involve the principal phases as described in Table 3.1, and certain phases might contain a greater number of steps than others depending on the nature and size of the project. As explained in Table 3.1, projects involving the development or purchase and implementation of information technology can have a more complex life cycle than other projects—including several stages—but they still essentially use the same tools and techniques to achieve project success. This does not necessarily mean that other types of projects are any less complex to manage.

The examples in Table 3.1 demonstrate the rational approach to the project life cycle, but this way of thinking about the phases of a project can mask a whole series of practical problems and difficulties that may later emerge, particularly when projects require significant change. As we explore each of the major project activities and tasks, this issue of the rhetoric versus the reality of projects, and ways of dealing with the gaps between the rational approach and the 'shadow side' (Egan 1994), will be addressed.

Table 3.1 Examples of project life cycle phases

Generic project	Health promotion project	Information Technology (IT) project
Initiate: Feasibility or needs analysis. This can be called the feasibility, analysis, strategy, conception, proof of concept or discovery phase. This is the phase that basically works out what you want to do and whether you can do it.	*Initiate:* Rationale, community needs analysis, literature review, action research	*Initiate:* Research, project scope, budgeting, acquiring capital funds, authorisation, finding a sponsor, specification development (technical, functional), planning of tendering process (expressions of interest), RFT (request for tender), vendor demonstrations, tender evaluation, contract with vendor, implementation planning study (undertaken by vendor), project initiation, planning workshops and functional, technical document production
Plan: Planning and design activities. This is sometimes referred to as the demonstration and validation, first build or preclinical deployment phase. In this phase you know what you want to do and you have to decide how you are going to do it.	*Plan:* Developing the plan, setting goals and objectives, defining tasks, timelines, resources, responsibilities and outcomes	*Plan:* Design of project management structure, technical architecture, product delivery, data migration, integration, implementation strategy, development, training strategy, testing strategy, issues and risk management strategy
Implement: Production, second build, construction or development phase. This is the difficult bit— making it all happen.	*Implement:* Hiring new staff, training existing staff, procurement of equipment, preparing material, organising and conducting workshops, seminars and project activities	*Implement:* Technical configuration, system configuration, system integration, system migration, software implementation, system testing (acceptance, user acceptance, regression), user training

		Go-live: Go-live schedule, operational readiness testing, process data migration, fix any rejected data, go-live support
Close: Turnover and start up, final or production and deployment phase. The product, deliverable or outcome is put into practice to see if it works. Evaluation is carried out to determine whether the project has met its aims, objectives and stakeholder expectations, and whether it did what it set out to do and is sustainable.	*Close:* Evaluation and review, often including a decision about whether to sustain the outcomes of the project as an ongoing part of the organisation's services or programs	*Close:* Transition from project status to support status, review outstanding issues, project review, closure

Differentiating projects and programs

In the health and community sectors there is a need to distinguish projects from programs or services. We have defined a project as a one-off effort, with clearly defined start and end times, tasks, management structure and budget, that is designed to achieve a defined goal. The term 'program' on the other hand, is used in two distinct ways. As applied in health and community services, a program is usually a service, intervention or set of activities that aims to meet a health or social care need. It may be ongoing, or have a defined operating period. Case 3.1 demonstrates how projects differ from programs in a community health service.

As shown in Case 3.1, when testing HEAL over six months with a small participant group, HEAL is being managed as a project, to be evaluated during and on completion. Once HEAL is offered routinely it is no longer a project, but a program that will be run regularly, using program management techniques to ensure that it remains effective and is delivered efficiently on a 'business as usual' basis. There are some real similarities between program and project methods, but it is useful to make the distinction. Projects are one-off activities with an end result

Case 3.1 Program and project in primary health care

Program: A community health service is planning to adopt the 'Healthy Eating and Active Living' (HEAL) program—an evidence-based type 2 diabetes prevention program—targeting people at risk of developing type 2 diabetes who live in the local government area. The HEAL program's main aim is to reduce the participants' risk of developing type 2 diabetes through lifestyle behaviour changes. The program helps them develop their skills, knowledge and motivation to achieve and maintain these lifestyle changes. The HEAL program runs over six months and is divided into two parts. Participants are supported and motivated to reach a weight-loss goal by adopting a healthy eating plan and taking part in moderate daily exercise. The program objectives include participants increasing their physical activity to five 30-minute sessions per week; developing a positive attitude to their own health; improving aspects of their diet (by 50 per cent); and improving their confidence in their ability to manage their health (by 60 per cent). Upon completion, participants are referred to local support networks to help them to maintain their improved lifestyle. The community health service is planning to run this program twice per year and to review it on an annual basis. Before implementation, the service would like to pilot test this program, to identify any implementation problems and to trial (for example) specific recruitment strategies and coaching methods.

Project: To recruit fifteen participants (aged between 45 and 55 and at risk of developing type 2 diabetes) for the HEAL program between May and October. The aim of the project is to test the program's capacity to reduce participants' likelihood of developing type 2 diabetes, by trialling and evaluating the success of the method in this setting. By the end of the six-month project, achievement of the program objectives by this group of participants will be measured to test whether HEAL can produce the intended benefits in this setting, and to identify any changes required for successful implementation of the HEAL program as part of the ongoing activities of the community health service.

(which may include trialling and refining a program or service); whereas health or community programs are types of service or activity—which may be ongoing or short term—through which the organisation enacts its health or community goals. As one senior manager we interviewed explained, projects are often used as a tool to trial an idea before a large investment is made in programs and services:

> ... [in this organisation] projects come out of a work plan or government initiatives and I think what one person would call a project other people would call program development. You might have a project that's about developing and implementing a new funding model, for example, as one sort of project but then you could have a project that was going to roll out national reform.
>
> *(Senior health manager)*

The other use of the term 'program management' in the project management literature is to mean 'a group of projects managed in a coordinated way' to obtain benefits not available from managing them individually (PMI 2008). 'Program management' is also used in a more general sense, to include both projects and ongoing business activities. For example, Roberts (2011: 14) refers to a program as a:

> management vehicle for progressing, coordinating and imple-menting an organisation's strategy, specifically by linking together an often complex combination of business activities and new projects, all of which are focused on the delivery of a defined business objective.

Project management methods

The objective of using a project management method is to ensure projects are successful, through the use of tools and techniques that enable projects to progress in effective, disciplined and reliable ways. A project management method is essentially an approach that can be used to help conceptualise and understand the tasks of managing a project to success, and how and when to use project management tools. Using such methods does not guarantee successful outcomes, but success is less likely without them. However, choosing a project management method is not always a simple task.

Experienced project managers sometimes give the impression that the use of a favourite model or method is the only way for projects to succeed. But in fact, our research confirms that there are several methods of project management in use in the health and community services sector. Many organisations use their own in-house tools and methods, a hybrid of methods or occasionally no method at all. While certain principles and methods are necessary for project success, in most instances there is no one best way, and no single recipe for success.

Our interviews with project managers and senior managers revealed the use of more sophisticated project management methods—for example, **'lean thinking'**—as compared with our earlier research. Examples of project management methods in use were PRINCE2®, Investment Logic Map, and Redesigning Care (based on the principles of lean thinking).

However, one fifth of interviewees reported some very basic approaches:

> we sort of project managed . . . in that . . . it's a defined piece of work we need a bit of governance over it. We need to write what we're going to do, we need some timelines and we need to know who is responsible for what. Now I think that's project management.
>
> *(Senior health manager)*

> If you're a good organiser and a good manager, having a governance structure and timelines and everything is normal practice anyway.
>
> *(Senior government manager)*

Others reported that their organisations didn't require a project management method, or expressed their belief that projects required longer timelines when an established method was used. The use of customised in-house approaches (based on modification of standard frameworks) was the norm, for reasons of conformity with the organisation's established practices and ways of thinking, and to simplify the task:

> Keeping the fundamental principles but to make them as simple and user-friendly as possible . . . and have a standard project

methodology. I just think we bind ourselves too much on doing the right thing by using [standard methods] every step of the way.

(Senior hospital manager)

Once you have to have an advisory committee and a stakeholder reference group and a board you have to maintain all that—you know, that's the other issue with project management, you don't want the management of the project to mean you don't have time to actually do the work because you're so busy managing all the governance and everything you've put in place. I see that a lot.

(Senior health manager)

The use of mandated project management methods was also seen as potentially bringing an unnecessary risk that:

if you were to have one project management methodology that required you to fill in boxes rather than think about what it is you're trying to achieve you could get people taking that path rather than thinking it through properly.

(Government senior manager)

The mixing and modifying of existing project management models and tools was achieved by consulting project staff, determining local need, finding common understandings and thus redesigning techniques to match requirements.

There was also some variation in practice in different settings. Some government departments and authorities had adopted a specific project management method such as PRINCE®, often with local modifications, and used it as a framework, a set of guiding principles for project management. Whether a model of project management is used can also depend on the source of funding. If the project involves a tender process or a consultancy, some standardised methods used by government may be stipulated as part of the funding arrangement, including methods of contracting, **tendering** and procurement, and rules of **probity**.

Examples of project management methods

Several proprietary project management methods are available and two of the more recognised ones, PMBOK® and PRINCE® are reviewed below. Many other methods are available in a multitude of textbooks and manuals on project management, but they vary in their relevance to the health and community services sector. We give more detailed consideration to these and other methods in later chapters.

A guide to the project management body of knowledge (PMBOK®)

Published by the US-based Project Management Institute (PMI), *A Guide to the Project Management Body of Knowledge* (PMBOK® Guide—4th edn 2008) is a widely used reference that encapsulates generally accepted project management knowledge and practices, and claims to be 'a recognized standard for the project management profession' (PMI 2008: 3). The PMBOK® Guide package includes a source guide for project management books. The project management knowledge areas described in the PMBOK® Guide are project integration, scope, time, cost, quality, human resource, communications, risk and procurement management. Rather than being a recipe book for successful project management, this publication is an excellent resource explaining theories and principles of project management, project processes and phases, and relevant tools and techniques.

We have drawn on PMBOK® throughout these chapters.

PRINCE® and PRINCE2®

PRINCE® (PRojects IN Controlled Environments) is a structured set of components, techniques and processes designed for managing any type or size of project (CCTA 1997). Originally developed for use in information technology (IT), it is owned by the Central Computer and Telecommunications Agency (UK), and it has been mandated in the UK public sector and is widely used (and perhaps often simplified) elsewhere. The PRINCE® method is a process-based model for the management of projects, and includes templates and tools that provide 'a framework whereby a bridge between a current state of affairs and a planned future state may be constructed' (CCTA 1997). The philosophy behind the PRINCE® model is that although every project is technically unique, by having a single, common and structured approach to project management the need to devise a specific approach for each project can be avoided.

PRINCE® provides an overview of project management theory, as well as practical methods for thinking about how the project fits into the organisation, how to go about planning and initiating the project, and managing the stages of the project. The PRINCE® package also includes templates that can be used as is or adapted—for example, a project brief, quality plan, business case, communications plan, risk log and end of project report.

Project management tools

Project management tools are used to assist project teams to achieve specific tasks. Common tools are Gantt and PERT charts and computerised scheduling and tracking tools such as Microsoft Project™ or Mac Project™.

Many organisations covered in our research had their own standard tools and templates for project proposals, plans, communication, risk management, status and variation reporting, and a few had implemented software to facilitate some project management processes, so it is useful to check what is available in the workplace. If this is not fruitful, it is worth looking a bit further afield. While the principles of project management are understood in some sections of the health and community services industry, a vast amount of information about the tools and techniques of project management is available in other industries, especially in engineering or IT fields. It must be said, however, that some of these more technical tools are limited in their usefulness in the health and community services environment.

Project management is an art, not an algorithm, and requires knowing when and how to use tools and techniques (Kliem 2007). Many will be ineffective unless they are supported by strong management practices, including effective negotiation, communication, leadership, use of alliances and networks, and change management methods. As described above, our research indicates that health and community services are generally using local adaptations of project management methods, and this also applies to tools.

Computerised project management tools and technologies

The general computerised tools we use every day are also useful in project management. These technologies include videoconferencing, the internet, GroupWare and network database management systems, the local intranet, scheduling software, voicemail and email. Webinars, blogs and online learning tools have the potential to add value as project tools.

There is also a wide range of project management software packages available to assist in the management of projects and in the establishment of an organisation-wide project management information system. But again, there is more to project management than just using project management software—it does not manage the project for you. The potential pitfalls in buying and using project management software include:

- the purchased software may never be used
- the software may be used for limited functions—for example, as a drawing tool, or for timekeeping or budgeting
- inappropriate or overly sophisticated software may be too unwieldy and too large to be useful
- detailed training may be required to use the software effectively
- the project manager may become too involved in the software, to the detriment of the project.

Microsoft Project is a commonly used project management product which enables the use of Gantt, PERT and critical path charts, milestones, project baselines, resource allocation and a work breakdown structure. Unfortunately, training in the software is sometimes the only training that would-be project managers receive. It is important, when evaluating project management software, to have a good idea of which tools would assist in the management of individual projects, and whether there is a need for a management system for multiple projects. Project management software, as with any other IT application, needs to be thoroughly evaluated in relation to the organisation's existing systems, software and projects. The process of evaluation and implementation of project management software is a project in itself.

The method or the tool?

There is a difference between a project method and a tool. The *method* is the practice of the activity; the *tool* is the mechanism by which it is achieved. For example, monitoring the project schedule is an important method of ensuring timeliness, and the Gantt chart is a useful tool for the task. It is easy to get carried away with an impressive array of tools, but it is important both not to lose sight of the underlying method and to choose the correct tools for success.

Some authors and managers believe that there is a technique or tool to cover any project management situation. For example, Kliem (2007) states that project management is all about tools, knowledge and techniques for leading, defining, planning, organising, controlling and closing a project. Others firmly believe that a good manager is also a good project manager; that project management is really a case of common sense based on experience; and that special tools and techniques do not necessarily add value. Project management methods may also be seen as a hindrance because they are too mechanistic, or as being of limited value in dealing with health and community organisations because they are designed for other environments. The balance is probably somewhere in the middle, in that formal project management methods have their place and are of particular value in some projects, but cannot of themselves ensure project success.

Project management resources

In this section, we present a short guide to finding project management resources which can both assist project staff to skill-up quickly and assist students of project management to find their way around the literature. These resources, many of them available free in libraries and from the internet, include project management textbooks, internet sites, databases, journals, templates, professional organisations and training courses.

Project management textbooks

A number of practical and useful project management textbooks are available, featuring varying amounts of jargon and technical complexity. There are not many texts that explore project management in health and community services (hence the need for this book). The following are suggested as good all-round project management texts that project managers (and students) might find useful when investigating project management theory or when initiating or managing a project:

- Billows, D. (2011). *Essentials of Project Management: Focus on using MS Project*. The Hampton Group, Inc., Denver, Colorado.
- Hartley, S. (2009). *Project Management: principles, processes and practice* (2nd edn). French's Forest: Pearson Education Australia.
- Kerzner, H. (2009). *Project Management Case Studies* (3rd edn). Hoboken, New Jersey: John Wiley & Sons.
- Lewis, J. P. (2007). *Fundamentals of Project Management* (3rd edn). Amacom, NY: McGraw Hill.
- Longest, B. B. (2004). *Managing health programs and projects*. San Francisco: Jossey-Bass.

- Martin, V. (2002). *Managing projects in health and social care*. New York: Routledge. Chapter 7: Estimating time and costs.
- Meredith, J. R. & Mantel, S. T. (2009). *Project Management: A managerial approach* (7th edn). New York: John Wiley & Sons.
- Office of Government Commerce (2009). *Directing Successful Projects with PRINCE2 Manual*. Norwich: The Stationery Office Books.
- Office of Government Commerce (2009). *Managing Successful Projects with PRINCE2*. Norwich: The Stationery Office Books.
- Phillips, J. (2006). *IT Project Management*. New York: McGraw-Hill Professional.
- PRINCE2 official textbooks at www.prince2.com
- Project Management Institute (PMI) (2008). *A Guide to the Project Management Body of Knowledge (PMBOK® Guide)* (4th edn). Pennsylvania: PMI.
- Project Management Institute, Inc.: Various textbooks on global standards grouped into 'Foundational standards', 'Practice standards and frameworks' and 'Standards extensions': www.pmi.org/PMBOK-Guide-and-Standards/Standards-Library-of-PMI-Global-Standards.aspx
- Rosenau, M. D. & Githens, G. D. (2005). *Successful Project Management: A step by step approach with practical examples*. New York: John Wiley & Sons.
- Verzuh, E. (2011). *The fast forward MBA in project management* (4th edn). Hoboken, New Jersey: John Wiley & Sons.

Project management journals

The leading journals dedicated to project management theory and practice are:

- *International Journal of Project Management* (Elsevier ISSN 02637863)
- *Project Management Journal*, Project Management Institute and John Wiley & Sons, online ISSN 19389507.

Most professional and management journals also carry articles about project management in their specific areas from time to time. These include *Australian Health Review, Harvard Business Review, Health Care Management Review, Health Services Journal* and the *Journal of Health Care Management*.

Internet sites and project management organisations
There are a large number of project management organisations with helpful websites. Many are dedicated to training in project management, while others offer services and tools. The following internet sites are considered to be key sites in their countries of origin:

- Australian Institute of Project Management (the peak body for project management in Australia): www.aipm.com.au/html/default.cfm
- Project Management Institute (US-based): www.pmi.org
- Association for Project Management (the UK peak body): www.apm.org.uk
- International Project Management Association (based in Europe): www.ipma.ch
- Project Management Institute China: www.pmi.org/About-Us/Customer-Care/China.aspx
- Project Smart 'Project Management Articles': www.projectsmart.co.uk/articles.html
- The Project Management Center: www.infogoal.com/pmc/
- www.projectmanagement.com a fun site directed primarily to IT project managers.

Project management skills and careers

Achieving good project outcomes depends upon good project management, and both the literature and participants in our research stress the importance of having the right person in this role. Simply applying project management principles isn't enough, because while project management may be a set of methods, it is also an art. The art lies in understanding what the project must achieve, and in being responsive to contingencies, open and flexible, aware of the situation (including tapping into your intuition) and able to deal with crises. Of equal importance are the ability to just get the job done and the persistence to keep the project moving on.

Project management skills

While larger projects may have a team of staff, it is often the case that a single project officer takes on the functions of both manager and team, frequently sharing the role of project manager with the person they report to. They usually need to negotiate with other staff for contributions of time, energy and support (and we note that this is true for almost all projects in one way or another). So even sole operators of projects need to pay attention to coordinating the work of others and motivating their (virtual) team.

Opinions differ about the importance of content knowledge for the project manager—that is, does it matter whether the manager has expert knowledge in the project's area of focus? For example, in a project that will amalgamate two pathology services, how important is it that the project manager has a scientific background? For a project implementing a new diabetes service, does the project manager need a clinical background? How important are general project management skills and experience in these settings?

Our experience and our research indicate that content knowledge is a distinct advantage, and that working familiarity with the culture of the organisation and the professional groups within it is almost essential. But project management skills are also essential. One research participant, a government project director, agreed that knowledge of the business was important for a project manager: 'You've got to have people who understand the business who can adopt these methodologies to fit within the business'.

Our conclusion is that content knowledge should be defined fairly broadly. For example, for a project that will develop a clinical service, knowing the clinical environment, and its culture and dynamics is important, but you don't need to be an expert clinician. For an IT project, you need to understand the IT environment, information systems (including knowledge of the software development life cycle) and technical concepts, but you don't have to be an expert programmer. On the other hand, where a potential project manager has great content knowledge and general management skills, but lacks project experience, some training, mentoring and support might bridge the gap. In large organisations, this expertise is sometimes available from the **project director**, or an executive with responsibility for strategy and innovation (and whose job involves significant project leadership).

When it comes to selection criteria and choosing the best person, the general principles for defining the required knowledge and skills for any job apply. Knowledge and skills should be specified in terms of competence or ability required rather than particular qualifications or backgrounds. Careful definition of the requirements, so that there is a balance between strong content knowledge and project management ability, is also important. General skills and knowledge requirements include some or all of the following:

- Leadership ability—in particular, creates and shares the vision for project success, and motivates the team and stakeholders
- Discipline and drive—demonstrates application to the task, takes responsibility, shows decisiveness, has the ability to work effectively at both strategic and detail levels
- Excellent communication and interpersonal skills—talks to the right people, influences others, builds consensus, makes the project visible, negotiates, lobbies for the project, can manage conflict
- Initiative and organisation—works independently, meets deadlines and ensures follow-through
- Technical project management skills—has know-how and experience
- Local knowledge—knows the working environment and has the ability to adapt tools and methods to suit
- Analytical and reflective—keeps their eye on the ball, understands risks, can read situations, is flexible and responsive.

All of these skills, attributes, experience and knowledge add up to a tall order when it comes to finding a suitable project manager, and it must be said that much of what is required of a project manager is only gained through experience—of projects, of workplaces and of people. Finding good project managers, especially those with the skills to deal with complex or large projects, is not necessarily easy. Participants in our research also thought that the softer or non-technical skills of project management, primarily the people (and political) skills, were of equal if not greater importance than technical project management skills.

Of course, no matter how experienced, competent, enthusiastic and intelligent the person chosen for the job of project manager may be, they cannot expect to operate effectively without support and cooperation from senior management, staff engaged in the project and the organisation at large (Lock 2007). Good project managers are not made or developed overnight. However, experienced line managers will already have many of the skills and attributes outlined above, and the skills of project management can be learnt (see the listing of formal training programs at the end of the book).

We saw some evidence that the strategy of developing promising project staff internally has greater long-term benefits than the option of buying-in project management skills. Some of the organisations we studied had taken a long-term view, and had worked to develop a project management culture or to encourage project management thinking throughout their organisations. They also invested in both formal training and informal learning opportunities for key members of their staff.

Project management careers

In the wider health and community services industry there is evidence of increasing demand for project managers and project officers. A scan of newspapers and internet employment sites shows that there are many opportunities at all levels and areas of the health and community services sector for fixed-term project positions for those with industry experience and qualifications. Contract and project-based employment arrangements increasingly suit employers in the current funding environment.

The two examples of advertisements for project staff in Figures 3.2 and 3.3 indicate the kind of jobs on offer in health and community services.

Figure 3.2 Ad for a hospital-based project manager

Project Manager—Hospital-based fixed-term part-time

- **Lead the implementation of the 'Extended Scope of Practice for Physiotherapists in the Emergency Department' project.**

- **Apply your Project Management, Service Evaluation and Research skills**

- **Work where your expertise is in demand**

An exciting opportunity exists for a Grade 4 Physiotherapy Project Manager to lead the implementation of the Health Workforce Australia 'Extended Scope of Practice for Physiotherapists in the Emergency Department' project at North Western Health. As the Project Manager you will work closely with the Emergency Physiotherapy Practitioners at Northwood Hospital, to adapt, implement and evaluate the model developed by the Lead Organisation, Mountain Health, to meet the local needs of the region. Leading service redesign, evaluation and reporting as well as facilitating research will play a key part of your role. In conjunction with the Emergency Medicine team you will be responsible for providing training, supervision and credentialling of the Emergency Physiotherapy Practitioner to extend their scope of practice, including the supply and administration of analgesia and diagnostic imaging. Collaboration, communication and education with departments across the region including Emergency, Orthopaedics, Radiology, Pharmacy and Allied Health will be essential to successful implementation. Postgraduate qualifications in Musculoskeletal Physiotherapy, or equivalent, would be advantageous.

Physiotherapists with a keen interest in this area are encouraged to apply. Employment is initially for 12 months with an extension for the term of the project until (date).

Figure 3.3 Ad for a community services program manager

Program Manager—Community Services

The Foundation is now looking to engage a Program Manager on a 12-month contract to pilot a national cyber safety initiative. Reporting to the General Manager Programs and leading a team of four project staff, the Program Manager will have overall project management responsibility for the development and rollout of a national pilot project. The appointee will develop and execute project plans including managing delivery to timelines, monitoring and reporting. They will conduct a market review and needs analysis, and establish and manage processes, training, relevant technology and a Helpdesk. Post pilot implementation, the appointee will conduct an evaluation and make recommendations for program improvements.

You are deeply experienced at leading and executing large projects or initiatives in the corporate, consulting, public or not for profit sectors. Ideally, you have a solid understanding of corporate sponsorship issues and demonstrate knowledge of contemporary cyber safety issues, particularly as they pertain to children and young adults. You have completed relevant tertiary qualifications and exhibit highly developed stakeholder management capability. Critical to your success will be your ability to think conceptually, while motivating and inspiring a team to ensure the effective development, delivery and evaluation of this important national pilot initiative.

There is also an emerging career structure for project managers. Larger organisations are appointing senior project managers to positions that require them to plan, acquire funding and coordinate a set of major projects. Sometimes the leader of the project effort (who may have the title 'project director'), is also the senior planning and development officer for the organisation and a member of the executive. Experienced health and community services project managers are also recruited by consulting firms to jobs that offer increasingly complex project management tasks and team leadership and management roles.

A career in project management can involve a number of roles. A larger project may include several categories:

- Team member
- Group leader
- Technical manager
- Project director
- Program manager.

There are many pathways to becoming a project manager in the sector. Many practitioners build their careers on achieving notable success when asked to take on a small local project. Experience is one requirement; professional development and formal qualifications generally follow for those who decide to specialise.

Project management seminars, courses and professional development

Courses, training and professional development in project management are offered by universities, project management organisations, consulting firms, technical and adult education facilities, and registered training organisations. Project management education is available by distance education, online, on site and face to face, although there are only a few tailored to the health and community services sector. There is no single recognised qualification in project management in the sector. This is mainly due to the fact that the majority of project managers gain project management skills and experience on the job; it is also due to the wide range of projects—from building hospitals to developing new models of care—that are undertaken. However, there are certificate, diploma and masters level courses in project management available through universities and further education facilities that provide the relevant skills, as well as the credentialing that assists in career development. See the listing at the end of this book for details on some of available project management courses in Australia.

Summary

- An understanding of the meaning of project management is important for the project manager in health and community services.
- Project management has a unique language, but many of the principles are familiar to experienced managers.
- The project life cycle is a useful model for thinking about and managing the phases of a project. It can also assist project staff to refocus and reframe the project if necessary.
- There are a number of project management frameworks, models, methods and tools that are of assistance in understanding project management concepts and theories. However, no single approach or method can guarantee project success.
- Project management software can be useful—and there are many good products available—but it does not substitute for leadership and sound management.
- Skilled project managers are in demand, and there are many valuable resources available to assist project managers, including books, internet sites, journals, seminars and courses.

4

The initiation phase: what do you want to do and why?

Chapter outline

Where do good ideas come from?
Getting to project goals
Goals, purposes, problem statements and benefits
    Project goals and objectives
    What are objectives?
Project scope and strategies
Turning ideas in projects
    Participatory approaches to developing project ideas
Planning and analysis methods
    Needs analysis
    Economic evaluation
    Literature review: using the evidence
In praise of opportunism
Responding to grants and tenders
Offering project tenders
Summary
Readings and resources

This chapter explains the first stage of the project life cycle—turning good ideas into practical project proposals. We start with the question of where ideas for projects come from. The chapter then explains the key steps to be taken in developing an idea into a project proposal that can be used to seek support, funding and approval, using methods and processes that work well in health and community services. The chapter addresses the question of how to get support for your project ideas, and concludes with a discussion of submitting applications in response to tendered projects or funding rounds, and contracting projects to consultants.

Where do good ideas come from?

Projects generally emerge from the combination of a community or organisational need—to solve a problem or take up an opportunity—and a good idea about how to meet that need. In our research we found that good ideas for projects arose everywhere, and that the process of emergence and capture of good ideas varied with the size and nature of the organisation and its approach to innovation and development. It is often the leadership group who identifies problems that need a project-based solution and then commissions project work. This top-down approach has the advantage of senior management support and therefore better access to resources. However, if the project requires change in the processes of service delivery, it may be more difficult to get staff further down the hierarchy to own and support it (this support is known in project management language as 'buy-in').

Good ideas also arise at other levels of the organisation. Discussions among colleagues—about problems that need solutions, or new ways of thinking about them—in team meetings, case conferences, at professional forums or in the tea room, are a common source. Sometimes projects emerge simply because someone thinks of a better way of doing something (or reads a success story from elsewhere) and lobbies decision-makers to test it out.

Other management activities, such as strategic planning or organisational needs analysis, often give rise to projects. Project ideas may be a result of external opportunities such as a new funding round, a call for tenders or a change in the law (for example, a new occupational health and safety requirement). Our interviews indicate that project identification is becoming a more proactive process, although several senior managers still saw this as a challenge:

... how are they identified? Sometimes by passionate people that come forward but I think we need a rigorous process to go out to the organisation and say 'okay, it's time'—like capital time, business time—time to identify what you think we should be thinking about over the next year project wise. Take it through the business planning and development process and use criteria and match it to that.

(Senior hospital manager)

Good ideas, then, depend on organisational strategic directions, individual passion and sometimes serendipity, as well as funding opportunities and good timing, in order to be developed into potential projects and, ultimately, be approved.

Getting to project goals

The first step in taking a good idea and turning it into a project is to define the proposed goals—what do you want to achieve? Our experience in practice and teaching as well as research has taught us that one of the most challenging tasks in developing a project is defining the goal in a way that lends itself to implementation and achievement. Case 4.1 illustrates the value of clear project goals. In health and community services, people often have a passion for their work and the energy and commitment to innovate, but if they are not clear on exactly what they are aiming for when they begin, the project is in trouble from the start. The general project management literature also stresses poor definition of what the project is trying to achieve as a factor in project failure (PMI 2008), and the people we interviewed emphasised overambitious goals as a big issue—it seems that we almost inevitably overestimate what can be done. One participant, a consulting manager, gave an example of trying to implement a large national project: 'we concluded that this is becoming increasingly difficult on such a grand scale and it might be better to do things in a more narrow focus'.

In the early stages of a project it can be difficult to take the step of turning a worthy aspiration into an achievable project goal, for many reasons. Sometimes it is simply lack of familiarity with the technical meaning of goals in project management, but it may also be due to conflicting priorities among staff designing the project or to problems in matching the team's goals to the requirements of the funding agency.

Case 4.1 From aspiration to project goal

Staff in a small community agency were interested in reducing tobacco smoking in young people, and they felt that this could be a major project for their service. After some investigation and some hard thinking about the resources at their disposal, they recognised that such a goal was too vague and too big, and did not enable them to define clear indicators of success. Based on their investigations, they defined a project that involved working with the peak tobacco control body and the schools in their community to ensure that high school students in their area had access to skilled support during a major citywide campaign about smoking (which involved television advertisements and an interactive computer-based information package). Their new goal was 'to ensure that high school students in our community have access to skilled support for avoiding or reducing tobacco use through their schools and teachers'.

They had not let go of their aspiration to contribute to reducing the health consequences of smoking, but they had committed to a focused, achievable goal—the first building block of a successful project.

Whatever the reason, the process of getting to a focused goal almost always forces greater clarity about strategies, timelines and the meaning of success. Now is the time, at the concept stage, to debate the need for the project, the evidence for effective responses, the project's relevance to the organisation or unit's strategic goals and the potential to gain allies and support. At this stage, debate about these issues can be enormously productive. Later on, when resources have been committed and movement towards the goal has begun, such debate can cripple a project's chance of success. Further on in this chapter, we explain how to use evidence and analysis to establish the value and validity of the goals—depending on the level of debate, you may need to gather the evidence early in the process.

Goals, purposes, problem statements and benefits

The general project management literature is clear that a project goal is a statement of what the project itself will achieve (Funnell 1997; McCawley 1997; Roughley 2009) expressed in concrete terms. But in health and community services it is not always so clear, particularly when projects are the basis for testing or implementing health and social programs.

Project goals are not statements of the reasons why you want to do the project. They are statements of what the project itself will actually achieve, in response to the problems or opportunities that the project will address. This is easiest to explain using an example from another sector.

The local government of a city built on both sides of a river needs to consider building a new bridge, because of increasing traffic congestion and consistent delays for traffic crossing the river. Bridges are expensive, so this is a serious decision. In considering whether and how to proceed, the local government authority undertakes traffic and engineering studies that estimate the benefits and costs of the project; they consult businesses and residents; and they measure pollution levels and so on.

Ultimately, they make a decision and, in this case, they decide to build a particular size and style of bridge in a particular place. Their *reasons* for building the bridge are basically to reduce congestion on the existing bridges and feeder roads and to enable traffic to flow more smoothly. These reasons can be stated in terms of *benefits* that can be measured—such as 'reduction in citywide cross-river journey times of five minutes on average during week days'. However, for the bridge builder, the project *goal* is much simpler—it is 'to build the bridge on time, within budget and to the required specifications'.

Applying this logic to the example in Case 4.1, the reasons for the staff developing this project include their commitment to improving the health of young people. The benefits if the project is successful will include fewer young people taking up smoking, and current smokers reducing or quitting their habit, as well as the proven long-term health outcomes that result. But the goal of the project is more modest. It will be achieved if the community agency succeeds in engaging with schools, teachers and students, and in offering skilled support and good resources to participants to the desired level (for example, the number of students who resolve to quit smoking, or not to start). Please note the implication of this way of thinking about project goals—while goals are expressed in terms of the things that can be delivered by the project, benefits usually accrue after the project is complete, and can't be assessed for some time.

In contrast, social and health programs are often formulated with an overarching goal that states the purpose of the program (which may be initiated as a project, but is essentially a new service or intervention). For programs, it is important to start with a goal statement related to health or social outcomes that will result if the program is successful and is sustained. Table 4.1 defines some important elements of the kind of analysis that gives rise to programs, and shows an example from the field of falls prevention.

These different frameworks can be confusing. The program approach may be required if your project is essentially about setting up or testing a social or health program. Clarity about the stages of decision-making and action can resolve the potential confusion. That is, the organisation can agree that the first stage should be making a decision as to whether to set up this program, based on a full analysis of its **program logic** (Taylor-Powell et al. 2003) or a similar model, including an assessment of needs. If the answer is that the program should be established, the work of designing a project to set it up can begin. We focus on project goals, objectives and strategies in the next section, and then explain some of the methods of using evidence to support project proposals, especially those that are about setting up or changing a health or social program.

Project goals and objectives

One of the fundamentals of project management is the principle that you first decide *what* you want to achieve, then work out specifically *how* to do it. There is of course an interaction between the 'what' and the 'how'—people always tailor their goals according to their means as well as finding the means to achieve their goals. But the principle remains, and the staging of project development accordingly is important: be clear about what problems you are going to solve or what needs to be addressed and what you want to do; *then* agree on how you're going to do it; and *then* get on with it.

Table 4.1 Goal, objectives and strategies for a falls prevention program

	Definition	Example
Problem statement	A statement detailing the main types of needs to be addressed and/or key problems to be solved by the program	High mortality, morbidity and costs associated with falls among high-care residents across ten residential facilities in a local council area
Program goal: anticipated long-term benefits	A statement about the broad and long-term change (desired outcome) that the program is working towards. The goal is what you ultimately want to achieve, to address the stated problem.	The reduction of mortality, morbidity and costs associated with falls
Program objectives: anticipated immediate/short-term benefits	Statements about specific and immediate changes that are needed for progress towards the goal. Objectives relate to the goal and are encompassed in the goal. They state what will be different as a result of the program and form the basis of strategies or actions.	• To increase at-risk residents' balance and strength by 20 per cent • To reduce the incidence of falls by 50 per cent • To reduce incidence of fractured neck of femur by 50 per cent • To reduce annual health-care costs for falls by $500 000
Strategies	A plan of action, designed to achieve the objectives, that describes how you are going to get the changes you want. Strategies are implemented through a series of activities and are best when based on evidence.	• To introduce a falls risk assessment method • To ensure all staff are competent in falls screening and prevention • To introduce a falls monitoring system • To reduce falls hazards in the facility • To ensure all high-risk residents are offered hip protectors

What are objectives?

Objectives, like goals, are statements of what you want to achieve, but at a lower level. If you are going to meet your goal, what are the main steps along the way—the parts that taken together will add up to achieving the goal? Project goals are achieved by fulfilling all detailed objectives. In other words, objectives are more specific and immediate changes that must be achieved in progressing towards the goal. Objectives in turn form the basis for strategies, and hence the activities or tasks by which the project is implemented. Table 4.2 gives some examples of an aspiration (or reasons for undertaking a project, and potential benefits), a goal statement and a statement of objectives for two projects.

As noted above, in many health and social programs, goals are closely aligned to the problems to be solved or the needs to be addressed, rather than simply being focused on the things that the project itself will achieve. For example, when the problem statement is 'high prevalence of androgenic anabolic steroid misuse among grade 10 male public school students in the local government area', the goal of the project may be expressed as 'to reduce the prevalence of androgenic anabolic steroid misuse among grade 10 public school students in the local government area'. The objectives will then detail immediate and small-step changes (measurable within the life of the project) that are needed in order to achieve the reduction in prevalence. These small step changes can be:

- improved self-confidence among students in saying 'no' to drugs
- increased parental knowledge and confidence to provide information and guidance to their adolescent children
- the development of positive attitudes about their appearance among the students
- the improvement of self-esteem.

The inclusion of these small-step changes is important as they will directly contribute to achieving the reduction in prevalence that is the longer term goal.

There are many ways to work towards a clear statement of goals and objectives: they can be established collaboratively through 'brainstorming' exercises; more information can be gathered to assess alternatives; and past strategies within the organisation can be reviewed with the involvement of key staff, managers and other stakeholders (such as health care providers, peer organisations or government departments).

Table 4.2 Examples of aspirations, goals and objectives for two projects

Project A: Social connections in the south-east	
Aspiration	To improve the wellbeing of people with mental illness and their carers in our region
Goal	To design and establish a service to reduce the social isolation of people with mental illness and their carers in the south-eastern region of NSW
Objectives	• To adapt the successful New Zealand 'social connections' program for our service system • To trial the program in one suburb and measure changes in levels of social isolation among participants • To evaluate the results and seek in-principle approval to implement the service across the region • (If approved in-principle) to finalise a plan for region-wide implementation, including the source of staff and financial resources required, referral protocols, and quality assurance for final approval by the Regional Executive
Project B: Surgical admissions pathway	
Aspiration	To provide better and more timely urgent and emergency care in a major regional hospital, by enabling urgent surgical patients who have been assessed elsewhere in the region to be admitted directly to surgical wards, without going through the standard emergency department (ED) assessment and queuing processes
Goal	To introduce a surgical admissions pathway for urgent patients straight to the receiving ward, and to test its capacity to reduce the overall length of stay for those patients and its impact on ED waiting times for all patients
Objectives	• To design the pathway in consultation with representatives of all relevant staff • To gain approval for trialling of the pathway • To implement the pathway for a period of six months • To evaluate the impact on length of stay and ED waits • To make recommendations to the surgical and ED divisions for longer term implementation

Source: Project B: Adapted from work by Mr Jason Cloonan

Later in this chapter we identify other techniques of gathering and assessing evidence that might also be helpful at this stage.

Project scope and strategies

The next major step is defining the size of the project and identifying what needs to be done to achieve the goals. Scope is a commonly used term for the definition of the reach of the project—what functions or systems are in or out, what target groups, what interventions and so on. If goals describe the focus, scope defines the borders. Generally, scope starts very broad, and is progressively narrowed as the practicalities of the project, and the challenges it must resolve, become clearer during the planning stage. Scope is usually defined when questions of who, what, where, when and how have been answered, and the project can then be given limits.

In a project, strategies are what you do to achieve the goals and objectives, or how you go about it. Strategies constitute a plan of action designed to achieve a specific objective and contribute to the broader goal (Eagar et al. 2001). Each strategy consists of a series of activities. Good strategies are:

- designed so that taken together they address the challenges the project is likely to face
- best when based on evidence of 'what works'
- feasible to implement, and affordable
- acceptable to stakeholders, and allow them to address their concerns
- consistent with organisational culture—style, values and skillsets
- consistent with relevant policies (organisational, industry, government).

For large and complex projects, **feasibility studies** and **economic evaluations** may be conducted to assess alternative strategies. Even in small projects, it is a good idea to check the available data for fit with the assumptions underlying your strategies. It is remarkable how often projects are designed to use strategies that can't work, sometimes precisely because of the problem they are trying to solve. For example, if the problem is poor access to cardiology services, it probably won't work to design an alternative pathway for access that depends on cardiologists doing more work. This may seem like an obvious mistake, but it is a real example.

Table 4.3 Objectives and strategies

Project A: Social connections in the south-east	
Objective	To adapt the successful New Zealand 'social connections' program for our service system
Strategies	• Establish a key service working group among all relevant service providing agencies and teams • Conduct a structured process for the proposal of adaptations; and discussion of the merits of each proposal • Prepare a draft 'Social connections in the South East' program for comment and sign-off by Regional Executive
Project B: Surgical admissions pathway	
Objective	To design the pathway in consultation with representatives of all relevant staff
Strategies	• Map the current processes of assessment, initial treatment and admission for the eligible patient group; design alternative processes and prepare draft pathway document using a working group of relevant staff representatives • Consult broadly with staff and other experts on the draft pathway and refer suggested changes to the working group for assessment, amendment of draft and sign-off

Generally, strategies can be designed to meet each objective in a project, as Table 4.3 illustrates for the projects introduced in Table 4.2.

Turning ideas into projects

Once the project goals, objectives, scope and strategies have been at least tentatively defined, much of the work has been done for an initial project brief. Many organisations in the sector have in-house templates or forms that enable staff with good ideas to formulate them into an initial proposal and seek in-principle support or approval to proceed to further development. These tools also aim to ensure that all the major questions are answered in a standard format.

The value of such an approach is, firstly, that staff are encouraged to articulate their ideas and think them through if they want to get support; and, secondly, that ideas can be assessed early on for fit with the strategic directions of the organisation and other important criteria. The **project concept brief** normally includes the following: a description of the problem or need or opportunity to be addressed and the potential benefits to be realised; the proposed project goals, objectives and strategies; the proposed timeline and possible resource requirements; and the relevance to the organisation's purpose and strategic directions.

These tools are variously called a 'project proposal', 'project brief', 'project scope' or 'project definition'. They sometimes vary between different parts of the organisation, to suit different kinds of projects. Well-designed templates can be a valuable way of guarding against sloppy thinking, as they assist proponents to identify whether their vision or good idea can really be translated into practical action. This tool can also be used by senior management to get an overview of what projects are being initiated within the organisation, for the purposes of prioritising, and also to monitor and manage the organisation's project portfolio. Like any tool, project templates can become bureaucratic impediments if they are poorly designed or inappropriately used.

The project proposal template shown in Figure 4.1 is designed to prompt proponents to think through the precise goals and deliverables, the required resources, the costs and benefits, the support from key stakeholders and the major components of work that will be required to take the project to successful completion.

If you are commencing this step, it's important to be realistic and to ensure that your project meets the organisation's criteria for support—not all good ideas survive the development and approval processes. In Chapter 2, we outlined the general criteria that senior managers often use to make these decisions (drawn from published studies and our research for this book). These criteria can be turned around and used as a guide for preparing project proposals that have a better chance of getting approval.

We suggest that staff preparing project proposals consider the following tips (not all of which might apply to any single project), and ask whether the project proposal measures up:

- Relate the project to achievement of the organisation's *strategic goals*, directly or indirectly
- Demonstrate (or imply) *good fit with culture* and values, existing and desired
- Write a *practical project plan that can be seen to be feasible*
- Marshall the available *evidence* that supports your idea
- Make sure the logic for your choice of *sponsor* for the project is clear and that any ruffled feathers are soothed

Figure 4.1 Project proposal template

Name of project:

Project sponsor: Proposer:

1. **Background to the project:** [Briefly explain the context and the problem or opportunity that gives rise to the project]

2. **Goals and objectives:** [What is the project aiming to achieve?]

3. **Rationale:** [Why should these goals be pursued through a project?]

4. **Scope:** [Briefly state the boundaries of the project. What is included and what is excluded?]

5. **Deliverables:** [What will this project produce?]

6. **Stakeholders:** [Who has power and influence? Who will be directly affected by the project? What are their concerns likely to be?]

7. **Timeframe and resourcing estimates:** [What is the likely duration of the project? Likely types and amounts of resources (labour and non-labour) required? What is the likely source of funding?]

8. **Risks and key assumptions:** [Identify all known major risks the project faces, and outline the major assumptions that may affect the project's viability or success]

Sign-off: _____

Proposer: _____   Sponsor: _____

Date: _____   Date: _____

- Deal with any *alliances or partnerships* that might be needed
- Demonstrate that required *skills* are available (or can easily be acquired)
- Make sure the *resource requirements* are manageable and well timed, and that the project cost is justified by the potential benefits
- Explain how the *results will be sustained*—that is, how the project outcomes can be embedded and continued in ongoing operations
- Demonstrate how this project will contribute to *organisational learning* and competence.

This checklist highlights many factors that can affect the chances of approval and support for project proposals. For example, management culture and culture of the organisation can be critical. If management is ambitious and proactive in trying out new ideas or service expansion, good project ideas will have a higher chance. This is not something that project proponents can change, but it is helpful to take them into account in shaping your project proposal. Timing, availability of resources and priority-setting are also important, as several of our participants pointed out:

> We have tried to have a coordinated approach to that so we have identified what we call priority projects ... that we're trying to get statewide coverage of ... but people like developing new little projects [and] it's very wasteful.
>
> *(Senior heath manager)*

In many cases, it takes persistence and belief—and commitment to achieving a high standard in the project—to get the project off the ground.

Participatory approaches to developing project ideas

As illustrated in Case 4.2, in health and community services it is a common (but by no means universal) practice for project ideas to be developed in a collaborative, participatory way. It is also good practice to ensure that consultation with stakeholders is carried out early.

Planning and analysis methods

There are three important technical planning and analysis methods that are commonly used in projects in the sector: **needs analysis** (or **needs assessment**), economic evaluation and literature reviews. Not all projects

Case 4.2 Using participation to develop project ideas

One large health service reported on its response to a funding program that had very clear objectives and addressed an issue that was a high priority for the organisation. The whole organisation was asked to identify potential projects or initiatives using a brief pro forma, which had been designed to collect good ideas while minimising the burden of writing the initial proposals. About 300 submissions were received.

A workshop with over 50 participants, including consumers and other external stakeholders, went through a process of bringing the 300 down to 12, with a great deal of grouping and melding of ideas through discussion. A 'village marketplace' was created through which people were able to add value or combine ideas, with ultimate prioritising through 'dotmocracy' (voting by allocation of coloured dots). The organisation's executive then endorsed the top 12 for submission.

While this process consumed a lot of energy, it generated a set of ideas that were well tested and broadly supported, using an overt, transparent process. The manager believed that the process was worth it for the organisation for several reasons, one being the need to ensure broad support for the projects that were ultimately funded and implemented.

will warrant the use of these methods, which can be time-consuming and costly, and require some technical knowledge and skills. However, if the project is complex or large in scale, these steps can be critical to test the merits of project ideas, and provide evidence for decision-making.

Needs analysis

The concept of needs in health and community services (and other areas of public policy) is used to determine the focus of interventions, services and programs. That is, services are seen to be worth funding because they can demonstrate that they are effective in meeting socially determined needs (because they produce the intended outcomes). Needs analysis (or needs assessment) is defined as an activity to develop a comprehensive understanding of the problems facing health or community service organisations and the needs of a particular group or community or population—this analysis is undertaken in order to identify the sorts of interventions or strategies that can solve those problems and address those needs (Eagar et al. 2001; Royse et al. 2006; Royse et al. 2009).

Bradshaw's classic typology of needs (Bradshaw 1972a, 1972b) can help in achieving a shared understanding of various ways of thinking about and measuring needs (see Table 4.4).

Staff in health and community services identify needs in many ways, often on the basis of their experience. However, when undertaking a formal needs assessment, other sources are required, and the 'big picture' of the service system, and alternative explanations of identified needs, must be taken into account.

> Usually we look at the evidence about need, we look at the evidence about implementation or what's been done before and whether it's shown to be effective, so [we need to ask] what are the right strategies to pursue, so we would always do that kind of background research.
>
> *(Senior health manager)*

A good needs analysis can be essential for generating support for a project. Needs analysis can be a critical step to turn a good idea into a project, and it can also be seen as a project in itself, depending on scope and complexity. As always, it is important to be very clear about the purpose and scope of the needs analysis; its intended users and what kind of evidence they will find convincing; as well as what will be acceptable and convincing for consumers and community and perhaps other stakeholders, like the local government authority.

Defining scope and focus of needs analysis

Well-designed needs analysis enables a systematic step-by-step approach to identifying and collecting relevant data and information. The first step

Table 4.4 Bradshaw's typology of needs

Felt need	What people identify and say they need. For example, pregnant women may feel the need for more information on childbirth and potential complications.
Expressed need	An actual request for services or programs—a felt need that has emerged as a request, either in the form of demand for services (people seeking the service) or through community action. For example, the need for a place to exercise in a local community may be expressed as a demand for exercise classes or the opening of a gym. Long waiting lists at the local GP clinics are a form of expressed need for more GPs to work in the area.
Normative need	Expert or professional views on what is needed, determined on the basis of research, professional opinion, value judgements or established standards. For example, the advisable levels of fluoride in water, the daily recommended allowances of nutrients in foods or accepted standards that specify the amount of open space for a given population.
Comparative need	Level of need is inferred by benchmarking against the volume of services or programs in comparable settings. For example, comparing access to supportive care and education for patients with diabetes in different geographic locations.
Latent or unmet need	This usually refers to a gap between known levels of need and actual take-up or availability of services or programs. For example, the gap between the number of diagnosed diabetics in a region and the number who access care, or the gap between demand for emergency admissions and the capacity of the local hospitals. This concept is useful for planners who need to predict the level of potential demand for services when designing new facilities.

Source: Bradshaw (1972a, 1972b)

is specifying the needs analysis questions. This may involve consideration of the following:

- Does the problem affect a particular population, community or group, especially a group that is disadvantaged in other ways?
- How prevalent is the problem—how many people experience it?
- How severe is it—does it cause serious debilitation or minor inconvenience?

- What is the service system capacity?
- What barriers and obstacles to change exist?
- Is this a study to argue for additional resources, or for the reallocation of existing resources to improve equity, or for reallocation of resources between different types of responses for the same need (for example, prevention versus treatment), or between different types of needs?
- Are there known effective interventions that should be included among the possible service responses (Hawe et al. 1990)?

It is very important to ensure you have developed the right questions to assist with the needs analysis design. Consider the two questions in Table 4.5 and note the different kind of investigations, scope and results that they imply. Limiting the scope, and focusing the questions, is important not only for managing workload but also to avoid or minimise the risks of raising false hopes or identifying issues and problems that are well beyond the scope of the organisation to address.

Table 4.5 Needs analysis questions

Needs analysis question 1: What are the gaps in follow-up services (within six months of treatment) for patients who have completed chemotherapy at City Community Health Service?
Needs analysis question 2: What are the specific needs of the patients (who have completed chemotherapy within a six-month period) that could be addressed by developing an integrated referral pathway between City Hospital Cancer Service and the City Community Health Service?

Gap analysis

As well as information about the number of people experiencing the problem that gives rise to needs for care or support or early intervention, information about gaps and potential capacity in the available service system—**gap analysis**—is also needed. Increased demand may result in unmet need, or it may be met with changes in the way that services are provided or with changes to the referral pathways among providers. That is, could the (potential or actual) gap be solved through more efficient services, through different kinds of services or through bringing together the responses of different service providers? For example, local Aboriginal and Torres Strait Islander people with cancer may approach health services later in the course of their disease than the general community, and the treating clinical staff may initiate discussions about the reasons for this and what could be done. Equally, community leaders may speak up and ask for changes in the way that members of the community are able to approach care providers or in the location and style of care.

This kind of problem requires both genuine engagement of service providers and community representatives, as well as good use of data to understand the causes and potential solutions, and their costs and benefits. There are four characteristics of current services that should be examined—awareness, availability, accessibility and acceptability—before decisions are made as to whether this is a case for a service improvement project or for new interventions or models of care. Measuring a gap in services to address the identified needs is as critical as measuring the identified needs.

Needs analysis methods

Once the needs analysis questions have been finalised, methods for collecting data and information can be decided upon, with priority given to reliable sources that can provide meaningful and valid answers to the questions. Data can be from secondary sources (that is, already existing data collections, perhaps requiring new analysis) or from primary sources, which usually means people. Table 4.6 gives examples of secondary and primary data and ways they are generated.

Table 4.6 Data types

Primary sources, requiring interaction with people	Secondary sources
• Focus group discussion • Community forum and consultation • Survey—email-based, web-based, telephone, written • Qualitative personal interviews	• Population data including demographic data, and social and health indicators • Epidemiological data such as disease distribution and onset • Service data such as numbers of patients treated and level of service provided, waiting list and waiting times (including 'did not attend' rates) • Organisational and administrative data (internal or external)

Organisations also conduct needs analysis for other purposes, such as analysing the need for a human resource development program (DeSimone et al. 2002). The needs identified through such a process may lead to training and staff development activities, but they typically also identify other types of needs—for example, to overhaul the way work is done, the way jobs are structured or the arrangements for staff car parking. Any of these identified needs might require the development and implementation of a project. And, if so, the detailed data gathered as part of the needs assessment will be a vital input to the project definition.

Needs analysis process

The usual steps involved in completing the needs analysis process are illustrated in Figure 4.2, using the case of a care or service need.

Needs analysis report

The production of a needs analysis report is the final step in needs analysis. A needs analysis report is typically structured along the following lines:

- Background and introduction
- Purposes of the needs analysis and needs analysis questions
- Needs analysis design and plan

Figure 4.2 Needs analysis process

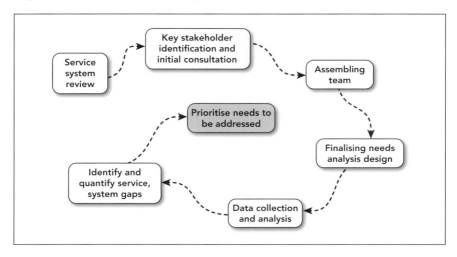

- Key findings (needs, problems, gaps, proposed interventions/solutions and so on)
- Discussion of findings and recommendation for further actions
- Conclusion and recommendations.

Needs analysis often results in a large amount of information, most of it very valuable, which can make it a challenge to prepare a succinct report with a clear summary of the findings and conclusions and a limited number of recommendations. This is where a tightly defined and limited scope of the analysis—specified at the beginning of the process—pays off.

Economic evaluation

Needs analysis may establish a convincing case for the merits of a particular project, but financial constraints are always present. An economic evaluation (Is it worth the costs? Will we be able to implement the results and sustain them?) may be needed to support the case for the project.

The reasons for undertaking this activity can be explained by example. Table 4.7 presents four questions for decision-makers. Consider the kind of information you might need if these decisions were up to you.

Typically answers to these questions are most strongly influenced by our estimates of the relative merit or value of the alternative course of action they pose. If there are sufficient funds, the decision is relatively easy—as long as the project is effective and produces the intended benefits. However, if funds are tight, economic considerations become

Table 4.7 Economic considerations

Question 1:
Should general practitioners monitor the blood pressure of every adult who walks into their offices?
Question 2:
Should a community service take on providing settlement help for newly arrived immigrants and refugees?
Question 3:
Should hospital administrators purchase each piece of new diagnostic equipment proven beneficial for fast and accurate diagnosis?
Question 4:
Should an organisation introduce a new system for monitoring adverse events that will cost $4.3 million dollars to install and $0.6 million each year to operate?

paramount. Are the benefits—for individuals or the population—worth the costs, as compared to other uses of that money? What if demand is higher than predicted? Economic evaluation is concerned with estimating the relative value of alternative options, and is designed to help decision-makers answer the following two questions:

- Is this service/program/intervention worth doing compared with other things we could do with these same resources?
- Are we satisfied that resources should be spent in this way rather than the other way?

The principle is that resource allocation decisions should maximise efficient use of those resources. In order to provide reliable guidance on this question for health or community service delivery, it is preferable to provide information on the related questions of:

- **efficacy**—can it work in testing?
- effectiveness—will it work in this specific environment and for this specific group of people?
- acceptability—will the people who are the intended recipients accept it?
- accessibility—will it reach those who need it?

Methods of economic evaluation of interventions or services include three main types: **cost-benefit analysis** (CBA), **cost-effectiveness analysis** (CEA) and **cost–utility analysis** (CUA). The difference between them can be confusing. *Cost-benefit analysis* estimates (in dollars) the costs and benefits of a given intervention compared with another intervention. In recent years, cost-benefit analysis has been criticised precisely because it reduces complex values, such as quality of life, to dollar figures. *Cost-effectiveness analysis* and *cost-utility analysis* express outcomes in non-monetary terms. CEA uses 'natural units' such as cure rate or reduction in the incidence of a disease. CUA attempts to express outcomes in quality-adjusted life years (QALYs) so that comparisons of benefit can be made between alternative conditions or service types. Table 4.8 provides some details of these three types of evaluation in terms of their measurements of costs and consequences.

Economic evaluation is normally carried out by health or welfare economists, who assume that resources are scarce and see economic valuation as an aid to rational allocation of recources. This type of evaluation uses concepts such as opportunity cost—achieving one sort of benefit at the expense of other benefits forgone—and marginal analysis—making

Table 4.8 Economic evaluation: measurement of costs versus consequences

Type of study	Measurement of costs	Indicators of consequences	Measurement/ valuation of consequences
Cost-benefit analysis	Monetary units	Single or multiple effects, not necessarily common to both alternatives	Monetary units
Cost-effectiveness analysis	Monetary units	Single effect of interest, common to both alternatives, but achieved to different degrees	Natural units (for example, life-years gained, disability-days saved, points of blood pressure reduction)
Cost-utility analysis	Monetary units	Single or multiple effects, not necessarily common to both alternatives	Healthy years (typically measured as quality-adjusted-life-years)

Source: Drummond et al. (2005: 2).

decisions on the relationship between the last dollar spent on a program or intervention and the benefit received for that dollar—rather than focusing on the average benefit of the program. Economic evaluation 'in theory allows decision makers to be more rational in determining which projects to fund or expand and which to cut or contract' (Carter & Harris 1999: 154).

Literature review: using the evidence

There is an increasing acceptance in health and community services that decisions, policies and practice should be based on evidence. From its initial establishment in the field of medicine, the concept of **evidence-based practice** (and policy- or decision-making) has been gradually accepted as a guide to policy development and health service management over the past two decades (Kovner & Rundall 2006; Shortell 2006; Cookson 2008; Head 2010).

For project proposals, this increasingly means referring to the relevant published research and policy documents, as well as to other more informal sources. Evidence may be scientific, but it is not limited to that (Lavis et al. 2005; Kovner & Rundall 2006; Liang et al. 2011). It includes:

- quantitative and qualitative research studies
- internal data, including reports, consultancies, evaluations and performance data
- examples of '**best practice**' in similar organisations or fields
- policy and management reviews, including auditor-general reports
- external consultants or expert opinion from acknowledged leaders
- information about stakeholder or consumer preferences (empirical or expert–opinion-based).

Thus 'evidence' is a broad concept. The search for and analysis of evidence is generally known as a literature review.

Literature review is a process of evaluating relevant information found in the literature and should describe, summarise, evaluate and clarify the evidence (Aveyard 2010). All work included in the review must be read, analysed and evaluated. Literature review can be an effective way of defining a problem; finding the current thinking on a subject; or assembling the evidence of effectiveness for a new method or technology, intervention or service. Literature reviews can assist agencies to avert misguided or even harmful projects that fail because they either do not meet a need or suffer from serious technical flaws in the way they are carried out. In other words, literature reviews can provide the evidence for decision-making about whether and how a project should proceed.

In Table 4.9, two examples (from the popular press and peer-reviewed research) illustrate why evidence is important in guiding service design.

Conducting a literature review: finding the evidence

The first stage in a literature review is finding the material, and this requires defining your subject area and knowing what you are looking for. Librarians use the Library of Congress subject headings when they are cataloguing books; these subject headings can be useful to help you decide where to focus your search. Using them, you can search library catalogues to find useful books, reports and journals, and get a good idea of the range of material available. The downside is that you will probably unearth a huge amount of material, much of it irrelevant and possibly out of date, as books in particular age quickly. Also, government reports, while essential

Table 4.9 Examples of 'evidence'

Warning to schools on misguided anti-suicide programs

Some school suicide-prevention programs are doing more harm than good . . . Poorly researched programs posed 'a very real danger' to vulnerable students . . . There are a lot of prevention programs run by well-intentioned but misguided community-based groups . . .

Source: The Age, 8 March 2003

Assessing cost-effectiveness in prevention

A study recently completed in Australia assessing the cost-effectiveness of prevention projects provided alarming evidence that a high proportion of prevention projects were not cost-effective, indicating a better approach should be adopted for the resources invested. Amongst the 121 prevention projects assessed, the research team found 47 out of 121 projects were not cost-effective with 3 projects even producing more harm than good.

Source: Vos et al. (2010)

for understanding directions and policy and so on, often present only the one viewpoint and can put a positive spin on activities and results that might be disputed in a more rigorous or independent analysis.

There are also citation indexes such as the Social Science Citation Index, and indexes of journals that your librarian can help you with. These can help you track down valuable journal articles and abstracts that might not appear in the main catalogue. However, perhaps the easiest and most efficient way of carrying out a literature search is to use electronic sources. These include the electronic databases for journal articles. Here keywords are more valuable than general subject headings—most databases will have their own lists of keywords to help you search. Some valuable databases include ABI/Inform, EconLit, ProQuest, Emerald for business and management, CINAHL, PubMed and MEDLINE (Ovid). Google Scholar can also provide a good place to start.

The value of journal articles and academic papers arises because they are often more current than books, and are subject to a peer review process intended to ensure some intellectual rigour. Research papers generally report on discrete research projects with clear aims and objectives, methods and analysis of results. The difficulty with journal articles is that sometimes they too are reporting on material that is a few years old. They can also be very technical and difficult to read and understand. Readers sometimes find that the problems investigated and presented in the articles are not of great interest to practitioners, and that the articles create more questions rather than providing answers. Moreover, findings and suggestions may not be sensitive and applicable to the local context in which the projects operate (Liang & Howard 2011).

Another key source of information is the **grey literature**—research that is unpublished or not formally published, and other sources such as government reports and websites. Examples of grey literature include policy statements and issues papers, conference proceedings, theses and dissertations, research reports, market reports, working papers and progress reports, maps, newsletters and bulletins, and fact sheets. This information may be circulated via your professional organisations and networks, and within the organisation where you work. Being unpublished does not mean poor in quality. Much grey literature is of high quality and value and often is the best source of up-to-date information on certain topics that may not yet have been widely studied. Using a search engine to find websites of government departments, professional institutions and non-government organisations is the starting point for accessing the grey literature. However, websites may have purposes other than to provide objective information. Their biases and their integrity need to be checked.

Finally, the thing to remember in literature searching is the importance of organisation—in other words, taking notes, keeping records (not only of the source but also of details like page numbers for easy reference later), highlighting important concepts and capturing interesting ideas and potentially useful quotes. There are several software programs (for example, Endnote™) designed to make it easier to record and cite references.

Making sense of what you find

The search of literature will unearth many references and sources well beyond the scope of what you are doing. Some will be obvious when you read the title and the abstract, and you will go no further; others you will have to read through to find whether they address your issue. Even if the paper interests you, you still need to judge its quality and relevance—that is, you need to critically appraise the evidence, and that requires some skill (Liang & Howard 2011). The essence of the process is to read each relevant paper, summarise the method and findings in a paragraph or two, and then write a few sentences summing up the impact of the results of the research, or the policy settings. The research centre 'Health Evidence', located at McMaster University in Canada, has developed useful resources including a standard step-by-step guide and forms to guide health professionals in searching and in assessing the quality of research (available at http://health-evidence.ca/).

After finding and assessing relevant evidence, the next stage is to tell the story of what you have found. This requires integrating the learning or the main findings from the sources you have read, and writing the answer to the 'so what?' question—that is, taken together, what does this literature mean for the scope, focus, design or conduct of the project (and the benefits or use the organisation may make of its results)? Thus the literature review may help to set the parameters for the project as well as establish what is known about the topic. The literature review should inform the reader about the weight of the available evidence, as the basis for your argument as to why your project is essential and/or valuable, and why it should be approached in a particular way. Two very useful books by Aveyard (2010) and Fink (2010) on understanding literature search and the literature review process are listed at the end of this chapter.

In praise of opportunism

We have focused in this chapter on the need to test project ideas for feasibility and relevance to strategic directions, and have advocated creative thinking and careful choices. However, the people we interviewed reminded us that there is also a place for opportunism, for several reasons. Sometimes an organisation needs to get runs on the board or build capacity and profile. Governments also respond to political issues, which may create opportunities. For example, if media attention is drawn to a problem that becomes a burning community issue—such as the use of drugs or inhalants by teenagers—governments will often respond by setting up a task force or establishing a project funding line to address the problem. Success then depends on the competence of project proponents to sell their good project ideas to the right people.

Responding to grants and tenders

In addition to seeking funds internally from the organisation, potential external funding sources should be considered at the early stage of conceptualising your project ideas. Seeking and securing funding is a skill in itself. There are sources of funding for projects for health and community service agencies, each with different criteria and requiring different approaches. Governments are important funders of projects, usually via a tendering or submission process. Potential project funds can also come from non-government sources such as trusts, foundations, charities and public donations.

When seeking external funds to support your project, the quality of the project proposal or funding application is critical. If resources allow, organisations sometimes contract consultants to assist with funding application development.

A tender is an offer submitted by interested bidders (organisations that apply or 'bid' to win the contract) to the agency commissioning the project (sometimes called the 'purchaser'), usually in response to a 'request for tender'(RFT), also known as an 'expression of interest' (EOI) or 'call for tender' (CFT). Some governments have promoted the competitive tendering process in many industries, including the health sector, in order to obtain competitive pricing for the provision of services. Hence, there are many opportunities for organisations to bid for and win contracts, often for ongoing service delivery, but also for projects. Government RFTs are advertised widely, both in the news media and on government websites, along with information about tendering policies and guidelines (for information on competitive tendering and contracting by government, see www.pc.gov.au/industry-commission/inquiry/48ctcpsa).

There are two distinct reasons for responding to a tender. Firstly, it may offer an opportunity to obtain funding for a good idea that has been under consideration for a long time—or for a variation of it. The other scenario is a more opportunistic one: a tender appears for something that has not been previously considered, or is perhaps not part of the agency's strategic directions but seems to bring other opportunities—and so a bid is made.

The questions and tips below are designed to help with the process of deciding whether to respond to a tender:

- Consider who is commissioning this project and why. Do you know what they are looking for?
- Do your homework, and use networks and contacts to find out as much background as possible.
- Always read the project brief/tender specification or funding guidelines carefully and always follow the instructions.

- Remember the application is for them, not for you—answer every question and respond to what they want to hear.
- Consider whether you are trying to fit one of your projects into someone else's project. If so, it might be difficult to achieve your aims (or even put in a successful bid).
- Consider whether the tender bid is realistic in terms of time and cost.
- Consider whether you have the necessary skills to carry out this project.
- Consider whether the roles and responsibilities are clear.
- Consider whether you have the support of senior management.
- Government contracts can be fierce about intellectual property (IP). Consider whether you will generate new IP or use your existing IP. If so, can your IP rights be protected?

Remember the organisation that has tendered out this project has done so for a reason—which was not to give you the opportunity to finance one of your pet ideas. The funder may not be impressed by the cheapest price, as one experienced senior manager explained:

> they may do a variation after they've got the job; I'm a wake-up to that, don't worry about that. I usually say to them at interview 'we've had five quotes, you're the cheapest by $400,000, what corners are you cutting?
>
> *(Senior government manager)*

Offering project tenders

For some organisations, projects mean involving consultants. This means that as soon as a project has been identified, it tends to go to outside consultants, either through a tendering process or directly to a particular company because of their successful track record.

Deciding to tender out a project can be a tricky decision, given the resources that are usually involved in preparing the specifications, and because of the tender process itself. Before putting out a project for tender, it may be useful to consider the following:

- Why is there a need to tender out this project? Is it because it is cheaper? Is there a lack of skilled staff? Or is it because the problem is best solved by an independent outsider with specific technical expertise?

- What kinds of people are needed to carry out this project? Can an external contractor feasibly achieve the required deliverables and outcomes?
- Are the skills and resources needed inside the organisation to manage the contract available?
- How long is it expected it to take, and what will happen if it takes longer?
- How much should it cost?
- Are there any hidden costs to the organisation that have not been budgeted for?
- Is there an allowance for the costs of contract management, and of responding to the consultants' needs for information and access to staff?
- Are the required roles, responsibilities, accountability and monitoring methods clearly described?
- How will this project be evaluated?
- Have any IP issues been identified and can they be resolved satisfactorily?

Essentially the tender process involves a number of steps, all necessary to ensure the best possible outcome and to fulfil the organisation's obligation to treat all bidders fairly. Key steps are:

- development of specifications for the project
- preparation of a request for tender (RFT) document
- call for expressions of interest and tenders
- establishment of a process for responding to queries from tenderers
- receipt and evaluation of tenderers' submissions
- notification of successful and unsuccessful bidders
- negotiation of the contract
- signature of the contract.

Public sector organisations are usually required to advertise tenders over a specified dollar amount, and usually they are advertised in newspapers or sometimes on websites. The tender process must follow the principles of probity (the integrity of the tender process), which include fairness, impartiality, transparency, security, confidentiality and compliance with legislative obligations and government policy.

The discipline imposed by the tendering process can be helpful in forcing clear specification and adherence to the project plan. However, it can also cause problems when genuine contingencies arise and specifications or methods and timelines need to be changed.

Summary

- Ideas for projects originate from both within and outside the organisation, with many instigated by government and other funders.
- Ideas for projects can be captured, evaluated and progressed using both formal and informal processes—for example, by using an 'ideas sheet' or a project proposal document.
- Participatory approaches to project development are more likely to enable effective stakeholder engagement, and can help to ensure the project is well designed.
- Projects need clear goals, objectives and strategies. Effort put in to getting them right in the early stages will pay off when detailed plans are developed, and implementation begins.
- Getting the project to 'in-principle' approval at the concept phase may require background work or research, including needs analysis, economic evaluation or literature review. These methods help to ensure that the need for the project is established, that it is based on good evidence and that it represents good value for money.
- Projects are often made possible by funding bodies who offer grants or invite organisations to submit tenders. Applying for funding involves significant work, but success is more likely if submissions and tenders are closely matched to the funder's requirements and preferences.

Readings and resources

Aveyard, H. (2010). *Doing a literature review in health and social care: A Practical Guide.* London: Open University Press.

Drummond, M. F., Sculpher, M. J., Torrance, G. W., O'Brien, B. J. & Stoddard, G. L. (2005). *Methods for the economic evaluation of health care programmes* (3rd edn). New York: Oxford University Press.

Fink, A. (2010). *Conducting research literature reviews: from the Internet to paper* (3rd edn). Los Angeles: SAGE.

Health Evidence at McMaster University: http://health-evidence.ca/

Muennig, P. (2002). *Designing and conducting cost-effectiveness analysis in medicine and health care.* San Francisco: Jossey-Bass.

5

The project planning phase: what will you do, and how?

Communications planning
Managing project change
Organisational change management planning
Planning project logistics
    The project information system
Planning for evaluation
    Types and frameworks of evaluation
    Benefits realisation
    Program logic
    Evaluation plan
    External or internal evaluation
    Data collection methods
Tips for conducting project planning
Summary
Readings and resources

Taking the time to properly plan a project, and developing a documented and agreed plan, can make the difference between project success and a troubled project that fails to deliver. Planning is the method by which the team works out how to make the project happen. A project plan addresses the 'what, who, how, when and at what cost'. It makes a project team more effective in achieving its aims and more capable of acquiring and using the right resources and methods. Good planning means selecting achievable aims, designing feasible means, managing the workload, identifying risks and issues, making the best use of everyone's talents and establishing the basis for good decision-making. Planning for evaluation of the project is also a key activity in the planning phase.

In this chapter, and Chapter 6, we explain the planning methods and tools that are most relevant to projects in health and community services. In this chapter, we focus on planning what needs to be done to achieve the project goals, and how it will be done. We bring together project planning methods with service planning and evaluation methods developed in the health and community services sector, and give a step-by-step outline for writing a good project plan. We also identify the issues that need to be resolved at this stage. In Chapter 6, we deal with three important technical planning methods—scheduling, budgeting and preparing a business case.

These techniques can be critical for larger and more complex projects (although we note that all projects require a schedule, and a budget of some kind). We have structured the planning material in this way so that readers can first get an overview of project planning as a whole, and then consider the more technical material in Chapter 6.

Why plan at all?

> Failing to plan is planning to fail.
>
> *(Attributed to Winston Churchill)*

Planning is working out what to do before action is taken (Rubin & Rubin 1992: 389). Every project management writer stresses that good project design and planning are critical to project success. The project plan is a blueprint for the entire project, and is the guide for future project activities.

Despite the good sense and obvious benefits of planning, there is often strong resistance to undertaking formal or detailed project planning. There can be pressure to get a project done quickly, and it can be very tempting to get on with the actual work of the project as soon as possible, and either avoid planning or pay it lip service only. As one research participant, a senior government manager, noted: 'people don't want to take the time or the discipline to think these things through properly'.

There are many reasons for resistance to planning, and they include the following:
- Planning can be difficult (it forces people to think—it requires negotiation, collaboration, consensus and decision-making)
- Many people believe that plans are a waste of time because inevitably plans change during the course of a project
- For most people, planning is not as satisfying as actually doing the work and getting quick results
- People lack the skills for planning
- A project plan can be seen as overly bureaucratic or as an organisational straightjacket rather than as a working tool (Maylor 1996: 46)
- Rational planning to determine the implementation or go-live date may seem to undermine the desire to 'name the date' that the team must work to.

Failure to start with a clear plan almost guarantees that your project will not be successful, because there will not be sufficient definition of what you are going to do or how you are going to do it. Without a project plan (addressing 'what, who, how, when and at what cost'), and without the plan being agreed to or signed off, it is likely that there will be general confusion, lack of common understanding, higher costs, and a lot of stress and discontent (Webster 1999: 14–15). Of course, the size and nature of the project will determine how elaborate the plan needs to be, and how much time and energy will be needed to prepare it.

It needs to be recognised that the time taken for planning and development can be anywhere up to a third of the total project timeframe and can equal the time spent on project implementation. The importance of good planning was reiterated by participants in our research, who identified that lack of (effective) planning directly contributed to project failure:

> Failure to plan mostly. Being overambitious, not spending the time being clear about what it is you're wanting to achieve.
>
> *(Senior government manager)*

> I think a lot of [problems] come back to that early planning, it's just so important to get that right at the beginning.
>
> *(Senior hospital manager)*

Senior managers are often tempted to 'name the date' when the project will be completed or will go-live, and will expect the project to be retrofitted to that timeline. In some instances there are imperative business drivers, such as the opening of a building. Often, however, the date chosen is more arbitrary—for example, the end of the financial year, or a visit by a politician or dignitary for a 'turning of the sod' photo opportunity. Unrealistic timeframes that are not based on a good understanding of the scope, tasks and resources will jeopardise the feasibility of the project. Compromise, or finding the middle ground, can be the answer in these situations, where the project manager will need to understand the logic and assumptions of the decision-makers, as well as inform them about aspects of the project that would need to be adjusted (such as scope or resources) to meet the required timeline. Sometimes, careful planning processes can solve these problems, as Case 5.1 illustrates.

Case 5.1 Naming the date versus planning and scheduling

The health service executive had just signed off an agreement with a web development company to develop a new public website for the organisation. It was announced to staff that the new website would be launched on 1 July, at the start of the new financial year (because the funding for the project needed to be spent by 30 June, the end of the financial year). But it was 1 April and the project manager had just been assigned the brief. A quick planning process involving the web developer, project team, project sponsor and key stakeholders identified the following schedule estimates:

- Initiation—establishment of project team, planning, steering committee (2 weeks)
- Design—review and approval of site map, look and feel and functions (4 weeks)
- Content gathering and update—gathering website content and review (6 weeks)
- Review and sign-off of new website design and content (2 weeks)
- Website programming by the vendor (6 weeks)
- Testing, review and launch (2 weeks).

By setting tight timelines and taking opportunities for activities to occur in parallel, the project manager determined that the project would take 20 weeks, with a launch date of 20 August. The project manager consulted finance staff, and devised a payment schedule with incentives for early completion of 'billable' work so that all expenses could be reconciled to 30 June. In this case, the project manager was successful in convincing the executive (partly because the logic of the plan was so clear), and it was agreed that the website would be launched in August.

The quality of the planning effort can also be crucial in the successful delivery of a project. The Victorian Ombudsman's investigation of ICT-enabled projects (November 2011) cited poor project planning as one of the key causes of the failure of the Victorian Health*SMART* ICT program, adding that 'the impact of many of the Health*SMART* time, cost and functionality problems encountered could have been avoided or minimised had [the Department of Health] adequately planned the project' (Victorian Ombudsman 2011: 70).

Planning methods

Because project planning is so critical in mainstream project management methods, there are many different terms in use and several models. All these models, however, are based on the rational planning framework. That is, planning proceeds in a logical order through the elements of the plan including rationale, goals, objectives, scope, strategies/approach, timelines, resources and evaluation. The jargon can be confusing, but the logic will be familiar. Table 5.1 outlines the processes involved.

Before we work through the steps and methods, we need to recognise that many newcomers to planning are sceptical about it, precisely because of the rational basis behind it. Working life is hardly ever as logical as the plan—people act in ways that are not imagined in rationales, goals and strategies, and may well set out to deliberately undermine or sabotage projects.

Sometimes circumstances mean that a project cannot 'start at the beginning', or that the rationale for the project has to be assembled after other decisions have already been made, or that the timeline is patently not achievable. Sometimes circumstances change during the life of the project. Sometimes the project team makes promises to stakeholders that it cannot keep, or the executive has another good idea that changes the project scope.

The value of planning can seem doubtful for **soft projects** (defined as complex undertakings aimed at intangible results). Most organisational change and service development projects have at least some of the characteristics of soft projects. That is (compared to building projects, for example), the objectives and scope are more likely to change after commencement, costs are more difficult to estimate and the logical relationships between activities are not as concrete (McElroy 1996: 327). However, experience with such projects (arguably the majority in the

health and community services sector) indicates that planning is especially valuable in conditions of uncertainty.

It is also important to remember that like the project life cycle (see
Chapter 3) planning is often an iterative process. For example, the project
may start with a clear plan, but the objectives might change when strategies are better developed in the early stages of implementation. New
possibilities might open up, or anticipated resources might shrink. There
can be frequent movement between planning and implementing activities,
particularly at the beginning of a project. Detailed planning for activities within the implementation phase—for example, testing, training and
go-live—may often be done just prior to the activity commencing.

Table 5.1 identifies the processes and activities of planning. Not all
the activities may be required for every project, but it is useful to start
with a complete list. Please note that some of the processes mentioned
below are explained fully in Chapter 6.

Table 5.1 Project planning process and activities

Components of the project plan	Activities
Project charter	Defining the goals, objectives and strategies
Scope and deliverables	Defining how big the project is going to be, what is within or outside the boundaries of the project, and what the project will produce
Project structures, governance and stakeholders	• Identifying the project sponsor and stakeholders • Locating the project in the organisation structure • Designing project committees and decision-making processes • Involving consumers
Activity definition, sequencing and timing (see Chapter 6)	• Development of the work breakdown structure (WBS); that is, the project tasks and activities, and the relationships between the activities • Estimation of how long each task will take
Schedule development (see Chapter 6)	Plotting project tasks against a timeline including project phases and decision points, deadlines, milestones and critical pathways

Human resources (see Chapter 6)	• Identifying the human resources required for the project • Building the project team
Resources, cost estimating and budgeting (see Chapter 6)	Defining and estimating the cost of the resources required for the project, and development of the project budget (see Chapter 6)
Risk and issue management	• Identifying what could go wrong (the risks), and the likelihood of it happening • Planning for contingencies and a process for resolving them • Planning for how project issues will be identified, documented and addressed
Project quality plan	Defining the quality standards to be met by the project outcomes and the systems for monitoring quality
Communication plan	Developing a project communication plan for informing stakeholders and reporting progress
Management of project change	Establishing change control and variation processes
Change management plan	• Identifying the change impact of the project, including the staff and processes that will be impacted • Developing a plan for how the change impact will be managed
Evaluation planning	Identifying how the project is going to be evaluated, what tools will be used, what data are required and how they will be collected
Operational planning	Establishment of the project tools and information systems

Source: Adapted from PMI (2008)

The key point is that hardly anything goes exactly according to plan, but having a plan helps you to deal with the chaos of real life and still get there in the end. Not having a plan is like negotiating the freeways of an unknown city without a map. You might be able to see the landmark you are headed for, but you are likely to end up somewhere completely different if you don't know the route.

The project charter

The project charter (or 'project scope', 'definition', 'statement of work') is the first key element and foundation of the project plan. If a project proposal has been prepared (see Chapter 4), it will provide the basis for the project charter. Essentially the charter could be described as the 'rules of the game' (Verzuh 2011: Chapter 4) by which the project runs. Everything else in the plan is based on achieving the project as defined in the project charter. Getting the charter right is a vital first step in planning, and this is where critical thinking about the project is concentrated and the project design is fundamentally set. When projects or a subset of tasks are undertaken by external consultants, the project charter will be a key part of the contract.

The key steps in preparing the project charter are:
- confirming/developing the goals and objectives
- outlining strategies and approaches
- defining the scope (that is, the limits)
- defining deliverables
- identifying key stakeholders.

For many ICT or information-system-related projects, the project charter and indeed the project plan may be developed as part of a process called an implementation planning study (IPS). An IPS may be conducted by the software or hardware vendor, in conjunction with the client, with a view to understanding the scope, deliverables (for both the vendor and the client), outcomes and risks of the project before commencement. The documented outcome of an IPS is often called the 'project definition' and becomes the basis for more detailed planning.

Strategies: how the objectives will be achieved

The simplest way to think about the strategies for a project is to consider each objective and ask: How will it be achieved? What needs to be done?

Some questions follow that may be useful to consider regarding strategy:
- Is this effectively an initial development and trial, and if so, how will it inform broader implementation?
- Will the project be staged or rolled out over time, or have a single implementation phase?

- For a staged implementation, which groups/areas would start first and what is the remaining order?
- What standards, policies or guidelines will be applied to the project?
- What approach will be used to engage key stakeholders/groups?
- What training and change management methods will be used?

The project charter should describe the strategies in enough detail for the project team, stakeholders and decision-makers to understand how the project will achieve its goals and objectives. Small, simple projects may not always need all three levels of goals, objectives and strategies. However, among these three levels it is the objectives that can occasionally be skipped, never the goals or strategies.

Project scope

Defining and sticking to the project scope is one of the cornerstones of good project management, as the scope statement puts some boundaries on the project (Verzuh 2011: Chapter 4). The research suggests that 'uncontrolled and undefined' project scope can be a major factor in a project failing to meet the desired timeline or budget, and that '**scope creep**' (unmanaged changes to scope—usually expansion) can undermine the success of the project. According to Hayes (2002), only one in five of all major projects actually meets schedule and budgetary goals. Many of the reasons for failure to meet the money and time objectives are found in the way the project was designed and how the boundaries around it were drawn.

Clarifying scope by having a scope statement in the project charter is the best way to safeguard the project. A scope statement should describe the major activities of the project and their limits in such a way that it will be absolutely clear if extra work is added later on (Verzuh 2011: Chapter 4). Often this is achieved by specifying what the project will *not* do (project **exclusions**), as these examples show:

- 'The system will be implemented in all Aurora Health campuses and locations, but excludes co-located services such as Rolling Valley Community Health and Eastern Dialysis services'
- 'Training will be developed and delivered to all ICU staff but will not include ongoing eLearning modules being delivered as part of the continuing professional development program'

- 'The project scope includes the piloting and evaluation of the new medication protocol, but not its implementation'.

The scope statement can also define where the project sits in relation to a larger or related project.

Defining deliverables

Consulting contracts often include a detailed statement of the products or outputs of the project that will be handed over to the client at the end of the contract. The deliverables are simply the answer to the question 'what will this project deliver?' and they might include a report, a piece of software, a process improvement, a training package or any product commissioned as part of the project. This concept can also be useful for internal projects, by forcing a clear delineation of the product or output in even more concrete terms than the goals or objectives.

Project governance

The project charter normally also includes a section outlining the proposed approach to project governance and decision-making, and the important task of engaging stakeholders.

The steering committee

Steering committees, advisory committees and reference groups can help to make or break projects. The term 'steering committee' (also known as 'project board' in PRINCE2® or sometimes called a 'project control group') usually implies some level of control and ownership over the project, indicating that the committee's decisions will literally steer the project in the direction the committee wishes it to go. Reference groups and advisory committees usually play a less hands-on role, providing advice and support and helping the project to work well. The design of the project committees, and their ways of working, will depend partly on whether the project is internally focused (for example, the reorganisation of care processes) or externally focused (for example, the development of an area health plan).

There are a number of critical issues in establishing the project management structure (PRINCE2® 2009: Chapter 4):

- Clarifying the role and decision-making capacities of the project committee
- Gaining appropriate representation on the committee

- Giving the committee authority to make decisions and commit resources to the project
- Identifying an effective chairperson who can facilitate interactive meetings
- Motivating members to persist with an often complex and demanding process
- Dealing with questions of confidentiality or conflicts of interest
- Ensuring community participation if relevant
- Securing participation by other parts of the organisation.

The PRINCE® method deals more extensively with project direction by a steering committee or board than many of the mainstream project models, in ways that seem useful for internal projects. Stakeholder management in internal projects has its own challenges—for example, there is often no defined 'client' to accept or reject outcomes. Individuals may have roles in both supplying inputs to the project and using its outputs, and the interests of stakeholders are sometimes seen as a kind of zero sum game—that is, one person's win is another's loss. In these circumstances, stakeholder paralysis is a real threat to projects that seek to change the way business is done.

In the PRINCE® approach, an empowered steering committee is chaired by the project sponsor (or executive in charge of the project). The committee takes the responsibility of signing off the various stages of the project and its final outcome. It makes decisions that are needed at this level all along the way, and acts as a sounding board for the project manager and team.

The committee is made up of senior representatives of the major stakeholder groups—that is, those who will use or work with the results of the project, and those who are required to deliver services or capacity to support the project outcomes. A deliberate distinction is made between 'suppliers' and 'users': the suppliers are asked to monitor costs and feasibility, while the users are asked to focus on functionality and quality. For example, in a project that aims to introduce a new information system into an emergency department, the IT department of the hospital will have a strong interest, along with emergency clinicians (medical and nursing), the health information and clerical staff of the department, and staff who manage the flow of patients into receiving wards (often called 'bed managers'). The IT department and the administrative staff would be asked to take the role of suppliers on the committee, and their vested interest is having a system that is efficient, and easy to maintain and support, is then formally recognised. The clinicians and bed managers are asked to take the role of users, and their interest in ease of use and quality of data is thus recognised. The health information staff might need to have a seat at both ends of this table.

In the PRINCE® approach (PRINCE® 2009), the duties of the steering committee or project board are to:

- be accountable for the project
- provide unified direction
- delegate effectively
- facilitate cross-functional integration
- commit resources
- ensure effective decision–making
- support the project manager
- ensure effective communication.

We suggest that the terms of reference of the committee are best considered at the planning stage, and developed and finalised in the early stages of implementation. Any potentially difficult issues should be dealt with up-front in a businesslike way to prevent them becoming really difficult and heated issues further down the track.

The role of the project sponsor

The sponsor or champion is somebody senior in the organisation who authorises the project and usually fulfils most or all of the following functions:

- Chairing the project steering committee or working group
- Acting as the supervisor of the project manager
- Ensuring that the project team has good access to people and resources across the organisation, as needed by the project
- Keeping the executive informed of progress, and ensuring their continued support
- Signing off (sometimes on behalf of the committee) on major decisions or variations as part of the project, and receiving the final report.

The sponsor may have been identified in the initiation phase of the project, with the tasks of defining the role and responsibilities and documenting them as part of the plan still remaining. If the project is contracted out, the equivalent role is generally played by the person who is 'the client' (who may be the person who signs the contract), and the functions are similar.

Identifying and engaging stakeholders

Stakeholders are the individuals and organisations who are actively involved in the project, or whose interests may be affected as a result of the project, or who may exert influence over the project and its results (PMI 2008). In the planning phase, the project team needs to identify the stakeholders, plan for their engagement and identify their interests and allegiances, which can affect the project. While this identification is not always easy, most projects will have stakeholders who fall into the following categories:

- Sponsor or champion—person or group who provides the finances as well as executive management support for the project
- Project manager—the person nominated to manage the project
- Customers or users—the people, groups or organisations that use or consume the project's product or outcomes
- Partners and allies—the organisations and individuals whose contributions or support is needed
- Performing organisation or department—the organisation or department whose employees are most directly involved in doing the work
- Project team members—the group performing the work of the project.

Once stakeholders have been identified, it is useful to consider the impact that a particular stakeholder group may have on the project, and how they will be managed. Stakeholders may have the power to veto or approve, delay, facilitate, derail or guide a project.

A simple map of the stakeholders is a useful planning tool that can help with preparation for active management of stakeholders' issues in the implementation phase, as represented in Figure 5.1.

To complete the mapping exercise, stakeholders are identified and categorised as to whether they are supportive of or opposed to the project, and rated for their relative importance—that is, the amount of power or influence they can exert on the project. Strategies for managing the way stakeholders engage with the project can then be developed, with the aim of minimising opposition and maximising support.

Figure 5.1 Stakeholder mapping

	Not important	Very important
Hinder	Problematic—need to be monitored	Antagonistic—need active strategies for management
Support	Low priority—keep on side	Champions—work with them

Involving consumers

Consumers as a stakeholder group need to be considered—consumer engagement can add value in several ways. The following factors are relevant to this decision:

- Will the project have a direct impact on care or services for patients/clients?
- Will the rights of consumers (for example, to privacy, or self-determination) be affected by the project?
- Are there issues of equity of access and appropriateness of service for population groups with special needs (for example, people with disabilities or mental illness, or for Aboriginal people)?
- Are there established advocacy or interest groups who can offer expertise and who might affect (positively or negatively) the success of the project?

The next question is to determine how consumers can be involved. While representation (for example, on steering or advisory committees) is one method, it isn't necessarily the best way. Focus groups, surveys and consultative groups (focused on the consumer perspectives and priorities) can make better use of limited time and energy.

Finalising the project charter

With the goals, objectives, strategies, scope, deliverables and key stakeholders defined, the project charter is now complete and can undergo a review and approval process. The approved project charter can be published to all who are associated with the project and then used as the basis for establishing the project and demonstrating management support for the project and the project manager (Verzuh 2011: Chapter 4).

The project plan

With the project charter developed and agreed, the remaining planning effort is directed at working out and documenting all the major resources and methods required to give life to the project charter. The length and complexity of the plan is primarily dependent on the size and scope of the project. Some organisations have templates and defined processes for the development of the project plan, and may stipulate what should be included in the document. Completed project plans can vary from about five pages to about fifty (or even more for large and complex projects).

The more carefully thought-through the plan, the more likely it is that the project will stay on track and the fewer surprises (or crises) there will be in the implementation and closing/evaluation phases. Energy spent in developing the plan to a sufficient level of detail, in collaboration with stakeholders, will result in greater understanding by all of what is expected of them as part of the project. In this way, much potential conflict can be avoided, or at least be identified and made more manageable.

The remaining planning effort and contents of the project plan address the following elements:

- Project structures
- Activity definition, sequencing and timing (see Chapter 6)
- Schedule development (see Chapter 6)
- Human resources
- Project resources (see Chapter 6)
- Risk and issue management
- Quality
- Communication
- Management of project change
- Organisational change management
- Project logistics
- Evaluation.

If the project is a small one, some of these headings might need only half a page in the project plan, but even small projects benefit from attention to each component. It is also important for the project plan to include any assumptions and dependencies that must be met before the project commences, or that may affect how and when it will progress. For example, it may be assumed that a government policy will be introduced by a certain date, or a project 'go-live' date may be dependent on a building redevelopment being on time.

The next area of planning—identifying the activities and tasks of the project—gets to the core of the work program, and the resources that will be needed to achieve it. The tools and methods for scoping and planning project resources (including the work breakdown structure, specifying tasks, estimating time and scheduling tools) are all described in Chapter 6.

Project structures

Planning for the location of the project within the organisational structure, and specifying its reporting lines and access to decision-makers, can prevent unhelpful project politics later on. The project manager's role will likewise be made easier if their place in the structure and the decision-making systems is clear and appropriate to the task.

Functional structures

There are a number of ways that projects can be structured within organisations, with no one right model. Functional structures (where the project is 'owned' by the unit or department most involved, the usual employer of most of the project team) have several advantages. They tend to have maximum flexibility in the use of their staff; individual experts can be utilised for many different projects; and specialists can be grouped to share knowledge and experience. However, a number of problems can also arise in this kind of structure. The project may suffer from a lack of focus and attention when it is competing with ongoing tasks, and the management of the unit may not be well placed to cope with project characteristics such as more urgent timelines. The project may require the unit to work with other parts of the organisation or another service provider in a way that is at odds with its ongoing relationships, or there may be an issue with staff not engaged in the project feeling exploited (Lientz & Rea 1998).

When projects within a functional unit come unstuck, the typical outcome is that they slip down the priority list and are delayed, downgraded or allowed to fade away.

The best predictors of success in this structure are that:
- the project is championed by the unit manager
- the team has authority to make decisions about the project

- the project deals with an issue that matters to the staff in their daily work.

The matrix system

The main alternative structure is the matrix system, where project staff are drawn from functional units, thus cutting across the organisation structure for the life of the project. The project manager reports to an executive or senior manager in the role of project sponsor, and the team members report to the project manager at least for the purposes of the project. The advantages of a matrix structure are that projects and project teams are given a strong identity within the organisation and resources are allocated accordingly. The downsides can include conflicts between line managers and project staff, undermining of the traditional organisation, conflict for staff working part-time on the project between their ongoing and project roles, and unclear roles and responsibilities (Alsene 1998). Case 5.2 illustrates the problem.

Case 5.2 Conflict between projects and operations

A health service established a project to implement national hospital emergency access targets within the organisation. The project manager tasked with planning and implementing the new access plan came from the quality and safety unit, while the project team was made up of representatives from the access management group, emergency department (ED) (medical and nursing), the heads of the surgical and medical units, the redesigning care team, IT and health information departments.

The project was sponsored by the executive director of nursing, and was given high priority, with an implementation period of four months. A matrix structure emerged by default rather than planning, with team members reporting to both their line manager and the project manager.

Great progress was made until the project required more time from the clinical staff than was anticipated (partly because of the short timeline). Releasing staff from shifts in the ED became increasingly difficult for the nurse unit manager, because of the needs of the daily operations of the department and the pressure on inpatient beds. In particular, the ED staff were caught between their daily responsibilities in the unit (some were accused of 'skiving off' and letting the team down) and effective participation in the project. There was also a common perception among ED staff that the project goal (to achieve compliance with four-hour ED admission targets for patients awaiting a ward bed) was purely a political target that was at odds with good patient care.

It became clear to the project manager and the executive that if the project was to stay on track, the resource costs to replace ('backfill') clinician staff time on the project would need to be covered. The project benefits to the ED staff and the organisation also needed to be better understood. It was time to revisit the plan, the budget and the stakeholder engagement strategy.

Risk management

All project management is risk management.

(Verzuh 2011)

Risk management is the means by which uncertainty is systematically managed to increase the likelihood of meeting project objectives (Verzuh 2011: Chapter 5). Risk management is essentially designed to answer three questions: What might go wrong? How will be it be handled? What can we do to prevent it, or reduce its likelihood? The related task of managing problems, opportunities and errors that arise during the project is generally known as 'issue management'.

All projects encounter uncertainty, and there is always the risk that something will happen to jeopardise the budget, the quality, the timelines, the stakeholder support and, ultimately, the achievement of the project's aims and its sustainability. Good planning includes a process for identifying project risks, understanding their potential severity and planning ways to respond if the risk becomes reality.

The aim of risk management is to control and reduce risk. The first step in the process is to analyse the project to identify the sources of risk. This is perhaps best achieved by consultation or a meeting with stakeholders to ask the critical questions and then create a risk management plan. What can happen to cause problems for this project? Will there be enough staff to cover the roster? Will the new equipment be delivered on time? Will industrial activity impact on the timeline? Will the software pass testing? Will there be a change of government policy or corporate leadership?

After defining the possible risks, including their potential impact on the project (that is, what is the result if the risk turns into reality?), each risk can be assigned a probability rating. Then a strategy (also called a **contingency**) can be developed to respond to the risks and reduce possible damage to the project and the organisation. To manage project risk effectively, a risk management plan should be developed as part of the planning process. This plan then provides the basis for the project risk register during implementation. Table 5.2 illustrates a risk management plan for the project of conducting a community survey.

Project risks are classified according to the likelihood of their occurring and the seriousness of the consequences or impact if they do occur. The likelihood may range from rare (for example, the chances of an earthquake) to almost certain (for example, the chances of minor vandalism in the car park), whereas the consequences may range from insignificant to catastrophic (for example, complete failure of the project or injury to patients). The risk level is assigned by plotting these two attributes of risk in the risk matrix (see Figure 5.2).

Verzuh describes various approaches to the issue of reducing project risk (2011: Chapter 5):

- Accept the risk—that is, choose to do nothing about it
- Avoid the risk—choose not to do part of the project
- Monitor the risk and prepare contingency plans
- Transfer the risk—for example, by taking out insurance
- Mitigate the risk—in other words, reduce the risk.

Table 5.2 Risk management plan example

Information	Description	Example
Risk	Description of the risk	Not enough community members are willing to complete the questionnaire
Risk impact	What is the impact of the risk on the organisation and/or the project if the risk is realised?	Project cannot effectively evaluate results of the survey, hampering decision-making about further project activities
Likelihood	How likely is the risk to be realised? (see Figure 5.2, 'Risk matrix')	Likely
Consequence	What is the severity of the consequence if the risk is realised? (see Figure 5.2, 'Risk matrix')	Moderate
Level of risk	The severity level of the realised risk when considering likelihood and consequence (see Figure 5.2, 'Risk matrix')	Moderate
Contingencies	What strategies can be put in place to respond to the risk to reduce the impact?	Gather information by alternate means; for example, focus groups or interview. Extend the survey.
Mitigation	How can the risk be minimised?	Involve staff that are familiar with the community and are influential
Risk owner	Which person or party has the responsibility for managing the risk and putting contingencies in place?	Project manager
Date logged	When was the risk identified?	April
Date of review	When was the risk last reviewed?	October

Figure 5.2 Risk matrix

Consequence / Likelihood	Insignificant	Minor	Moderate	Major	Catastrophic
Almost certain					
Likely					
Moderate					
Unlikely					
Rare					

Level of risk			
Low	Moderate	High	Extreme

Source: Prince2® Complete Document Template Version 1.0 3/4/00 Rational Management Pty Ltd

Once risks are understood, it is possible to identify contingencies—the 'what if' issues—and plan the response. Capital building and engineering projects always include a contingency allowance—that is, money set aside for unforeseen circumstances, usually about 10 per cent of the total cost. Projects in health and community services are often budgeted to the last penny, with no capacity for a contingency allowance. But even if adding an actual contingency allowance is not possible, there is usually a way to slip in some flexibility or some discretionary resources. If something goes wrong, resources allocated to another component of the project could perhaps be shifted without impacting on the core objectives; or some potential slack in the project timelines could be taken up; or the scope could be squeezed by cutting back on non-core elements.

As part of contingency planning, it is important to plan for an escalation procedure. To '**escalate**' means taking the project issue or issues higher in the organisation in order for them to be resolved, or implementing the next level of action required to overcome an identified risk.

Issue management

During the course of the project, problems, situations, opportunities, questions and errors can arise which are generally referred to as 'issues'. An issue can be defined as a problem or obstacle that the project team does not have the answer to or the power to resolve (Verzuh 2011: Chapter 5). Examples of issues could be delay in the supply of a project resource, a policy conflict exposed by the project, a key stakeholder either leaving or joining the project or any unforeseen situation not dealt with in the project plan. An issue log enables issues to be documented when they arise and thus provides the basis for assigning responsibility and ensuring the issue is addressed. It also establishes a record of how the issue was resolved or managed. The contents of a simple issues log are described in Table 5.3.

Table 5.3 Issues log

Issue ID	Unique identifier, usually a number, assigned as each issue is identified
Description	What is the issue and what is the impact if it is not resolved?
Assigned to	The project team member (or project manager) responsible for pursuing resolution
Date identified	Date the issue was originally added to the log
Current status/ Last action	The date of the last action, a description of the action, and the current status of the issue. Leave all the action/status lines in the log as a record of how the action was pursued. Keeping closed issues in the log is one form of project history.

The quality plan

Every project aims to reach a standard of quality in its outcome, at the least in order to be 'fit for purpose', and perhaps to meet external standards (for accreditation or other benchmarks) or to fit with the quality systems of the organisation. The project charter is again the source document for quality planning. What are the standards that each of the major deliverables or outcomes must meet? Are there process standards that apply (for example, 'consultation with unions is conducted in accordance with the organisation's formal agreements')? Who needs to be satisfied with the quality achieved?

Each project will have unique specifications, standards or criteria that need to be met. For example, a new information system for patient location search in a hospital might require an average response time of three seconds or less; a new strength and balance program for older people might have to achieve a high standard of safety. These requirements provide the elements for the project's quality plan. A simple quality plan for an emergency department project (introducing a new patient management system) is shown in Table 5.4.

Table 5.4 Quality plan for emergency department (ED) patient management system

Quality of outcomes	Measurement	Who accesses
• The flow of patients through the department is efficient and safe • The information needs of clinicians are met • Administrative staff can meet their workloads with current staffing levels	• Meets specifications for timelines and continuity of care • Meets specifications; no losses of information currently available • Workload of new systems is at worst equal to existing	• Directors (medical and nursing) of ED • Senior medical and nursing staff representatives • Administration manager
Process and indicators	**Measurement**	**Who accesses**
• Patient care is not disrupted during implementation • Staff are consulted and engaged in changes affecting them	• No adverse impact on patients is recorded during implementation • Meets organisational change agreement standards	• Directors of ED • Human resource consultant

Communications planning

Inevitably, almost all aspects of projects rely on effective communication—from policy decisions to meeting times. A breakdown in communication can be a project showstopper and is worth spending time on in the planning phase.

A communication plan is the written strategy for getting the right information to the right people at the right time (Verzuh 2011: Chapter 4). All the project stakeholders will need information on a more or less regular basis, so even a simple plan outlining who requires the information, what information they need and when they need it, is useful. A simple communication plan might look like the one outlined in Table 5.5.

Table 5.5 A simple communication plan

Stakeholder	Information required	Frequency	Medium
Sponsor	High-level cost, quality, problems and proposed solutions	Monthly	Written report and meeting
Sponsor	Risk escalation	As necessary	Phone, email
Project team	Detailed schedule, problems, news, coordination information	Weekly	Meeting and status report
All interested parties	Occasional news of the project	As and when required	enewsletter

As part of a communication plan, a standard format for reporting progress to stakeholders will help enable rapid and consistent communication. A template for a project **status report** (including communication plan reporting) is provided in Chapter 7 (see Figure 7.5). Also think about how other reports and communication can be as timely as possible. Consider paper reports, regular meetings, newsletters, email updates, intranet notice boards, message boards and blogs. A major project might employ non-formal communication strategies, as illustrated by Case 5.3. A useful principle when planning communications is to err on the side of more rather than less, as it is difficult to overcommunicate!

Managing project change

Projects never unfold exactly as planned, no matter how good the planning has been, and variations (or **variances**) are a normal part of project implementation. At the planning stage, it is important to anticipate the need for variations and design a process for identifying, documenting and managing project change. This is called project change management, as distinct from organisational change management (see the next section).

There are a number of formal tools for managing project change and they can be adapted to suit the needs of the project and the style of

Case 5.3 The Friday Facts

The project manager for a multisite project published a one to two page electronic update every Friday for 52 weeks— inevitably known as 'The Friday Facts'. It was sent by email to all interested people in five collaborating organisations spread over several cities and towns. The information was factual, the tone was casual and the layout was informal. Everyone who contributed was added to the email list, and the support staff appreciated being included and informed of the 'big picture'. For the recipients it was an easy way to keep up with the project, and it also contributed to overcoming the problems of distance in this complex project.

the organisation. PRINCE® and other frameworks call for a register or log of changes and a process to formally request changes to such aspects of the project as scope, timelines and deliverables. Such a register records the following for each change: the problem/change title, originator, date notified, project manager approval date, sponsor/client/steering committee approval date, implementation notes and, if relevant, change to the project completion date.

Organisational change management planning

The challenge at the beginning of a project and in the planning phase is to imagine what the organisational impact of the project will be, so that it can be effectively planned for and managed. There is a common but erroneous perception that change management is simply a matter of explaining the benefits of the project to those affected as part of the communication or training, and that sustainable change will result.

The change impact of a project may be significant for specific individuals, for a particular role and for the organisation as a whole. During the planning phase the focus is on anticipating the impact of change, or how it is going to be identified later, so that it can be managed effectively. For projects that entail significant change in the way services are delivered, or the way business processes are conducted (for example, implementation of an organisation-wide information system), process mapping and review during the planning stage may be needed to identify the change impact of the project.

'Process mapping' (or 'business process review') involves mapping workflows and information flows, sometimes using flowcharting software like 'Visio™', to document current and future processes. For example, when implementing a telemedicine service, a number of workflows (processes) for the doctor, nurse, allied health and administrative staff may be affected, including booking of the appointment, scheduling of the clinician time, documenting the consultation and billing.

It may not be necessary to conduct a full business process review in the planning phase, but simple high-level workflow mapping can assist in identifying several aspects of the impact of change. These include who will be affected, and whether their role or responsibilities will change, as well as the location of their work and how they will carry out a process. For example, in the introduction of electronic pathology test ordering, major change in the workflow for clerical and courier staff is likely. Workflow mapping will also indicate current versus future state—what is changing, what is staying the same and what will no longer be done—and will quantify the magnitude of change, in regard to what decisions will need to be made, and what policies will need to be reviewed and updated.

The project plan should include the strategies that you will use for identifying, quantifying and managing the organisational impact of the project, including change impact statements, business process review and policy review, as well as communication and training.

Planning project logistics

The project will need some systems for its own operation, and the physical resources to do so. The project plan should address the establishment processes and the required equipment, including information systems.

The following checklist highlights key issues:

- Is the project visible and identifiable—does it have a name or logo?
- Should the project be officially launched?
- Does the project have a home?

- Is there adequate space allocated for project team meetings, for workspace for project staff and for storage of project documents?
- Do you have the necessary resources, such as computers, access to photocopiers, fax machines, telephones and stationery?
- Is the project manager known and identified as being the project manager?
- Is the project manager the main or the only contact, and do people know how to make contact with the project?
- Is there an agreed process or expectations for formation of the project team? Will staff be identified and asked to join the project or will they be seconded or recruited externally? (Be aware of the lead time to form the team—it can sometimes take months for staff to be released and become available to work on the project.)

The project information system

A vast array of information can be generated during the life of a project. The documentation or data might include both hard and soft copies of the project plan, training program, variation requests, progress and status reports, budget papers, scope documents, meeting minutes and agendas, WBS, Gantt and PERT charts or schedules, contracts, policies, discussion papers, invoices and purchase orders, correspondence and workshop reports.

Regardless of the size of your project, the plan should include a system for dealing with data generated by it and with the information needed to manage it effectively. You may need to set up shared file directories that can be accessed by all the project stakeholders and team. Early planning can also enable the learnings from the project to be held and shared more effectively across the organisation, and contribute to future project success.

Planning for evaluation

Because each project offers a unique opportunity for learning from experience, evaluation is always of potential benefit. This can be a simple process, and doesn't need to be a whole research project in itself (although sometimes that is warranted). Evaluation needs to be planned for and built into the project at the planning stage, even for small projects—that is, the evaluation needs to be planned in advance, and starts while the project is actually running.

An evaluation provides answers to the questions 'did we do what we set out to do?' and 'is this going well?'. It also enables the lessons of the project, both good and bad, to be learnt and applied to future projects and programs, and provides an opportunity to reflect on outcomes, processes, organisation and methods. Evaluation can assist in completing a change process by consolidating both the evidence for the change and a common understanding of what it means. Evaluation can be a powerful method of building cumulative knowledge for later projects.

> Good project management is about reflecting 'How are we going? What's going wrong? How come that didn't work? How can we fix that?' but you would do that as part of [the project implementation]—and then when you finished you would all come together and say 'let's apply some hindsight' and we look at what we would have done differently—but that's part of the project management process.
>
> *(Senior health manager)*

Evaluation is a process by which we decide the value or worth of something by observing, measuring and comparing against an established criterion or standard (Hawe et al. 1990). Project evaluation can help monitor how your project is going, determine whether the project is making a difference, help to identify its strengths and weaknesses and assist in finding new strategies to improve the next project. Evaluation also provides information to support the continuation or extension of a project, and can be used in demonstrating accountability to funders and community members (SACHRU 2012).

Project evaluation is a process that will help the project team to review:
- how well the project is doing or has done
- how well it has achieved its goal, objectives and strategies
- what worked well, what didn't, and why
- whether there were any unintended outcomes
- what can be learnt from the project to improve practice and inform other projects (SACHRU 2012).

Types and frameworks of evaluation

Evaluation is usually classified into three types: process, impact and outcome (or summative) evaluation.

Process evaluation

Process evaluation measures the effectiveness of the strategies and methods used in the project, and the skill of their execution. We have already described some of the ways that project management practices (such as issues logs) build-in a requirement for consistent evaluation of progress, change and corrective actions. These are all part of process evaluation in a project.

A well-developed project plan effectively includes milestones, standards and criteria for assessing the processes of the project as it unfolds. Giving people real time feedback on what is happening can also enhance the project's chances of success.

Impact evaluation

Impact evaluation measures achievement of the project's goals and objectives—that is, it focuses on the short-term impact. Impact evaluation can also assess unforeseen and unanticipated outputs or outcomes, whether beneficial or detrimental.

Impact evaluation can be a simple procedure. At its most basic, the question is 'did we achieve the goal of the project?'. For example, if the goal of the project was to install a new system or process, the question is 'does it work?'. For some projects, this may be all that is done, and all that the organisation needs. But the impact evaluation questions for larger or more complex projects require more thought, and the project manager may need to choose or design **evaluation indicators** to make the impact of complex changes measurable. For example, in assessing the impact of a new model of care that requires nurses to work differently, sick leave levels may be an excellent indicator of real acceptance of change, to complement data on the level of compliance with the new method.

Outcome evaluation

Outcome evaluation measures the longer term achievements of the project. Impact and outcome evaluation both assess the effects of the completed project, but over different time periods (Hawe et al. 1990: 103). However, outcome evaluation is virtually impossible in the timeframes that apply to projects.

See Case 5.4 for an example of evaluation in the community setting.

Case 5.4 Evaluation in the community setting

A community health service had a request from a local general practitioner (GP) concerning the needs of an increasing number of Afghani women attending her surgery. She felt that their needs were largely social and emotional rather than medical and asked, 'Could you do something for them?' The agency met with the women's unofficial interpreter, and after much discussion set up a project to establish an Afghani Women's Health Program in the area. The project had three major objectives: firstly, to identify the health needs of Afghani women; secondly, to develop strategies to meet those needs; and thirdly, to raise awareness among other service providers in the area.

Discussion groups were held, resources were collected, and an Afghani Women's Health Forum was conducted, with invited speakers addressing important cultural and health issues. Other activities followed. Service providers in the area took part, and were successfully engaged in broader responses to the needs of the group.

The project was evaluated in a number of ways. As the project leader said: 'We first of all asked the question "Did we do what we set out to do—that is, did we establish the program?" The answer to that question was clearly, "Yes". Second, we collected data on the numbers of women and service providers attending all the activities, and we collected demographic data about the range of women attending— age, education, etc. Third, we asked for feedback from all participants in our activities through both participant feedback sheets and group discussion. Finally, we involved the Afghani women in decision-making about future activities, thus reflecting on what we had done and identifying what worked and what didn't. In this way we carried out both impact and process evaluation—we just did what seemed logical.'

An outcome evaluation of the project—that is, of its contribution to the better health of the women involved—was not possible, because the timeframe and the complexity of measuring health outcomes were beyond its scope. However, the project had both unforeseen and longer term impacts. For example, the women identified a whole range of issues as important to their health, such as housing, immigration, work and education, which went well beyond the issues the agency had initially considered. The women also organised among themselves and became very involved in local housing issues. One woman went on to open her own restaurant, actively supported by the others.

There was also an impact on service providers, who were made aware of the group's needs and priorities. They realised that some of their normal practice should be changed if they were to meet the needs of such a group. This realisation led to a series of cultural awareness projects in some of the mainstream agencies.

But there was another way the staff knew that the project had been a success. 'When they came to hold their meetings they filled the place up with laughter, colour, food and good energy. That good energy lifted the spirits of everyone else in the place—hard to explain in evaluation terms but easy to see and feel in practice.'

Benefits realisation

Another way of considering project outcomes and evaluating project success, particularly in relation to ICT projects is **benefits realisation**. A benefit can be defined as a net positive change in outcomes. The preparation of a benefits realisation plan (which effectively sets targets) and its formal use in the governance of the project is a way of increasing the chances that the benefit will actually be delivered (NSW Government 2009). Put simply, a benefits realisation plan is a tool to make sure you actually get the intended benefits originally planned for your project (NHS Institute for Innovation and Improvement 2008).

The implementation of clinical information systems and electronic medical records (EMRs) is often funded on the basis of the benefits that they will deliver. For example, for electronic ordering of pathology and radiology tests, one of the expected benefits would be a reduced number of inappropriate or duplicate tests ordered. For electronic prescribing, the expected benefits would include a reduction in medication errors. Benefits can be bankable (they can enable dollar savings, for example in consumables or space) or non-bankable—in the form of productivity gains (for example, time savings) or improved patient satisfaction. It should be noted that benefits are often not realised until some time after the project has been completed, and realisation plans often monitor benefits over a three-to-five-year period.

PRINCE2® includes a benefits realisation framework, which has been used in major ICT projects by the National Health Service (NHS) in the UK. According to the NHS, the value of focusing on benefits realisation planning is that you can track whether intended benefits have been realised and sustained after the end of the project. It also helps to ensure a clear signposting of who is responsible for the delivery of those benefits (NHS Institute for Innovation and Improvement 2008). Like other evaluation planning, a benefits realisation plan is often developed early, at the same time as the business case, and updated in the planning phase. A benefits realisation plan (NSW Government 2009) contains the following information:

- The key outcomes (considered a benefit) of the project
- The benefit type (bankable, productivity gain)
- Baseline and target measures to be achieved for each outcome (the benefit)
- The expected delivery schedule for each benefit
- An overview of the monitoring capabilities required to measure each specified benefit, along with details explaining how each capability will be delivered
- An explanation of the risks that may threaten the achievement of each benefit and how the threat will be handled
- The outcome owner.

Program logic

The program logic model is a method of planning and evaluating programs that is often used in the social, health, environment and international development fields. It is usually presented as a diagram, showing the relationships between the program goals, the required inputs and processes, and the intended outputs, impact (short-term results) and outcomes (long-term results). Its use requires the 'theory' (or logic) of the program to be made explicit, including the causal relationships between the elements.

While the program logic model is not often cited in the general project management literature, it is used for projects that develop and trial a new intervention or activity. Its advantages are the focus on clarifying the assumed cause and effect relationships (thus making it possible to test them) and the presentation of the overall logic of the program in a single diagram. The outline of a program logic model, and how it relates to process and outcome evaluation, is shown in Figure 5.3.

The program logic model is often used in project evaluation. It helps to determine what will be evaluated (based on an agreed understanding of the elements and their causal links), what to measure and what indicators to use. Most importantly, it helps the evaluators to analyse the reasons for success or failure, by focusing on where the necessary cause–effect relationships may not have been viable or valid.

A program logic model for a project does not replace the detailed project plan. Rather, it enables the logic of the intervention to be made explicit and provides the basis for an evaluation plan.

Figure 5.3 Program logic and types of evaluation

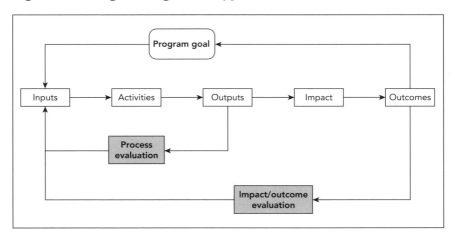

Evaluation plan

Part of planning is to determine how and when activities and milestones need to be reviewed (sometimes known as **tracking** in project jargon). The planning process, in conjunction with the tracking process, provides a practical, workable method to evaluate where a project stands. While the project goal and objectives are the bedrock for evaluation, the quality plan can also provide key elements. An impact evaluation plan should outline the standards, targets or outcomes against which the project will be measured; how the measurement will be made; and who will be involved. A process evaluation plan should outline the questions of interest and specify the stages at which they are to be considered, how and by whom. Table 5.6 shows an evaluation plan for the surgical admissions pathway project introduced in Chapter 4 (Table 4.2).

External or internal evaluation

'Insider evaluation' is carried out by the project team themselves with input from the key stakeholders. For the people involved, participation in evaluation assists in the process of finishing and moving on. Insider evaluation has the benefit of the participants' intimate knowledge and understanding of the project. It can encourage the development of critical reflection skills and assist in embedding these skills within the organisation itself. However, insider evaluation might be viewed as biased and therefore invalid or of less value than evaluation by others. And it might be less rigorous, since participants often want their project to look good and will dwell more on the positives, perhaps downplaying the negatives (Wilson & Wright 1993: 5).

Evaluation is often carried out by 'outsiders', perhaps a group of skilled specialists in a particular method or approach (for example, economic evaluation). Outsider evaluation is often seen as more credible but it is also more costly and is likely to be used only for larger projects. The benefits and limitations of insider versus outsider evaluation are described in Table 5.7.

Data collection methods

Some writers have criticised the use of traditional 'scientific' approaches to evaluation in health and community services, arguing that they are not appropriate for projects influenced by complex social and political networks and uncertain causal relationships (Pawson & Tilley 1997; Chen 2010b; Wadsworth 2010). They argue that realistic or naturalistic and interpretative methods are more valuable. These approaches often include quantitative data, but generally emphasise qualitative methods including interviews with key players, direct and indirect observation, focus groups and case studies.

In reality a range of methods and data collection techniques can be employed. This is likely to include 'hard' or quantitative data such as occupational health and safety or workforce statistics, and data on performance as well as the softer, more qualitative approaches. As Patton (1990: 9) argues:

> There are no rigid rules that can be provided for making data collection and methods decisions in evaluation. The art of evaluation involves creating a design and gathering information that is appropriate for a specific situation and a particular policy-making context.

The important point is that the project evaluation design is included as part of the project planning phase, so that the right information can be collected in the right way for that project as part of its implementation.

There are many different methods that can be used to collect information for evaluation. These include:

- analysis of records (attendance, admission, demographic details)
- surveys (mail, email)
- interviewing individuals (face to face, telephone)
- interviewing groups (for example, focus group discussions)
- documentation (journal/diary, log, progress reports)
- triangulation (combining data from different sources and methods to enrich analysis and insight).

Tips for conducting project planning

There are no magic solutions for overcoming the difficulties in conducting project planning and estimation. But some things can help:

- Seeking advice from colleagues with relevant expertise
- Consulting management and stakeholders early to ensure support and shared understandings of limitations and constraints
- Learning from the experience of other projects—many evaluation and case studies are available both online and in hard copy
- Committing yourself to targeted training
- Contracting professional project planners or consultants to provide support and advice.

Table 5.6 Evaluation plan for the surgical admissions pathway project

Goal: To introduce a surgical admissions pathway for urgent patients straight to the receiving ward and to test both its capacity to reduce the overall length of stay for those patients and its impact on emergency department (ED) waiting times for all patients.

Impact/goal achievement evaluation

Objective	Questions	Measures
Participative pathway design	Was the pathway well designed? Was it accepted by relevant stakeholders?	• Conformity with evidence for safety and quality • Sign-off by steering committee (and date)
Approval for trial	Was approval given?	• Approval to implement by relevant management (and date)
Implement for six months	Was the new process used for at least six months?	• Date of commencement and of review or closure
Impact on length of stay and ED waits	Were six months of data collected? • Was LOS reduced? • Were ED waiting times reduced?	• Acceptable data quality for at least six months • Reduction in LOS (statistical measure) • Reduction in ED waiting times >4 and >8 hours
Recommendations	Was a report, including recommendations, prepared?	• Report accepted by decision-makers as adequate for informed consideration (and date) • Recommendations considered and decision made (and date)

Process evaluation

Process	Questions	Method/measure
Pathway development	Were staff representatives satisfied with the pathway development process?	Discussion at meeting of representatives with a manager not involved in the project, using questions prepared by the team; notes of 'bests' and 'worsts' for representatives and overall level of satisfaction
Stakeholder management	Were staff representatives satisfied with the project overall?	
	Was the change managed well?	Analysis of change management process and challenges prepared by project team; discussion at final steering committee meeting; analysis amended and finalised.
	Were other departments (including the information division) satisfied with the project process?	Discussion with representatives of information services, finance, bed managers and so on; comments noted and compiled.
Communication	Were stakeholders well informed about the project, its progress and the nature of changes?	Inclusion of questions about communication in all methods above
Governance	Were decision-making and leadership of the project effective?	Discussion at steering committee meeting and with executive, by the project sponsor; notes prepared including 'bests' and 'worsts'
Close and handover	• Was the project closure adequate? • Was handover effective?	Review by team with project sponsor and representatives of surgical wards, ED and other departments involved in operation

Source: Adapted from work by Mr Jason Cloonan

Table 5.7 Insider versus outsider evaluation

Insiders doing the evaluation	Outsiders doing the evaluation
Benefits • Can have a deep understanding of project and its context • Likely to develop trust with staff and community groups involved • Part of the organisational structure • A way of developing evaluation skills, critical reflection • Less costly *Limitations* • May not have time to devote to evaluation • May lack skills in evaluation • Harder to be objective	*Benefits* • Bring an outsider's perspective • Can be viewed by funders as providing a more independent evaluation • Can provide a fresh look at the project • Provide evaluation expertise and experience from other evaluations • Can free up more time for the doing of the project *Limitations* • Greater cost considerations • Can have less knowledge of the project and organisational and political environment • Not part of normal organisational structure • May require time to develop trust among staff and participant

We noted at the beginning of this chapter that reality hardly ever works out in the precise, rational way that planning methods seem designed to achieve. This is not an argument against making a logical, detailed plan, but it does point to the need for skilled management and flexibility. Expecting the unexpected is the only possible outlook for project managers. In the next chapters we move to project management in action, and discuss how project teams manage what happens when the plan meets reality.

Summary

• Project planning is the critical success factor for projects and the project plan is the central pillar of project management.

• The rational planning approach involves the development of achievable aims, objectives and strategies in a logical order, even though reality hardly ever works that way.

- The foundation of the project plan is the project charter, which defines scope and strategies as well as aims and objectives.
- The other elements of the project plan detail how the project charter will be implemented. They include project structure, the work program and resources, planning for risk and quality, communication planning, change management (both project and organisational), project logistics and evaluation planning.
- Project governance—in other words, committees and decision-making processes—can provide important methods for managing stakeholders as well as for coordinating the advice and inputs the project needs.
- Risk and issue management planning involves identifying what might go wrong, what will happen to the project if it does, how likely it is to happen, what contingency allowances can be made, and what approach to take to each major risk.
- The quality plan specifies the standards that the project's outcomes must meet, and how their achievement will be monitored.
- Project logistics include getting the project established (office, name, logo and so on), the information systems the project will need and the communication plan.
- Monitoring and evaluation are critical for effective projects and the plan should include a method of evaluating the success of the project.
- Two proven approaches to evaluation currently in use for projects are benefits realisation planning and assessment, and the program logic model.
- Even after writing a great plan, expect the unexpected.

Readings and resources

Project management guidebook: http://www.thoughtware.com.au/documents/method123-ebook.pdf

Project planning: http://en.wikipedia.org/wiki/Project_planning

Project management tools: http://www.mindtools.com/pages/main/newMN_PPM.htm

Risk management planning:
http://www.wikihow.com/Develop-a-Risk-Management-Plan

Project Issues Register template: http://www.egovernment.tas.gov.au/_data/assets/word_doc/0012/77898/Project_issues_register_template_and_guide.dot

Project communications template: http://www.projectmanagementdocs.com/templates/communications-management-plan.html

Benefits realisation framework: http://www.archi.net.au/documents/resources/hsp/benefits/guide/benefits-framework.pdf

Benefits realisation plan: http://services.nsw.gov.au/sites/default/files/Benefits%20Realisation%20Plan%202011_0.doc

Program evaluation:

Centers for Disease Control and Prevention (US) evaluation site: http://www.cdc.gov/eval/resources/index.htm

South Australian Community Health Research Unit Planning and Evaluation Wizard: http://som.flinders.edu.au/FUSA/SACHRU/PEW/index.htm

6

Planning tools: scheduling, budgeting and the business case

> **The project business case**
>   **Writing a business case**
>   **What about projects with no positive business case?**
> **Summary**
> **Readings and resources**

In this chapter, we focus on planning the timing, activities and resources needed for projects—the core of the work program—and the technical tools that make it possible. Some of these tools may be unfamiliar to staff working in health and community services, but they are worth knowing as they can be powerful aids to demystifying the when, how and how much questions that can seem unknowable without good tools and techniques. We also explain the related strategy of developing a business case. The more general tasks of project planning are addressed in Chapter 5.

Work breakdown structure: tasks, sequencing and timing

A journey of a thousand miles starts from beneath one's feet.

(Lao Tse 1963: 125)

The tools and methods for specifying the tasks, sequencing and timing of the project enable the project manager and the team to:
- document all the tasks and activities that have to be completed
- identify the resources required to complete the tasks
- see the relationships and dependencies between the tasks
- track progress against a timeline, and identify milestones within the project
- identify how long the project will take and any deadlines (or critical points) within the project.

Project strategies cannot work unless there is a clear action plan, with the necessary staff, resources and equipment at hand. It is sometimes useful to pre-test strategies, perhaps through a pilot or feasibility exercise. For example, if you are developing a questionnaire to use with a particular group, it could be pre-tested on a small sample to discover whether the questions make sense, flow in a logical order and extract the kind of information you are hoping to find. If you are planning to carry out a project that involves a specific group—whether they be medical specialists or the mayors of local towns—it is often useful to speak to just a couple of representatives first, to explore ways that the group as a whole might think about an issue. This way you will be informed about and prepared for the likely attitudes and issues you may encounter. These activities should be identified in the planning stages and written into the plan.

The activities and tasks of a project need to be defined and broken down into manageable chunks. The simplest way to do this is to start with the goals, strategies and deliverables identified in the project charter. You can then break them up using subheadings and expand on them in a list format. In project management terms this is called creating a **work breakdown structure** (WBS). The WBS is 'a tool that the project team uses progressively to divide the work of a project into smaller and smaller pieces' (Kloppenborg 2009: 142) and is a mechanism for 'breaking down' the project goals into manageable tasks to allow estimation of project time and costs to take place (Kliem et al. 1997). The concept of the WBS was initially developed by the United States Department of Defence in 1962 (Hamilton 1964) and has been widely used in all defence services since, spreading gradually to other fields (Haugan 2003). The process of building a good WBS forces significant issues to arise early rather than later in a project, and also provides the basis for estimating the time and cost of the overall project. In fact, the WBS is a powerful tool for expressing the scope of a project in a simple graphical format.

There are many techniques and rules of thumb for developing the WBS that can help with sizing the tasks and defining the relationships between them, as well as with other technical aspects. Some tasks require specialised knowledge and skills, some need to be managed independently and others require teamwork. Identifying and detailing the tasks can be difficult, and the ideas will probably flow faster if it is done by the team or a working group rather than an individual. WBS provides a clear picture of the sequence of all project tasks to be completed, and enables the team to estimate the time and intensity of tasks, and to develop a better understanding of who can best get the work done.

Key components of WBS

A WBS is a hierarchical structure with a single 'box' at the top representing the whole project, as shown in Figure 6.1. The project is then divided into components fitting into the lower levels of boxes in the WBS diagram. It apportions the entire project into logical chunks of work, which are then subdivided and arranged in the right order (Hill 2010).

The second level of the WBS is the deliverables—the products or outputs that together represent everything the project must achieve (Hill 2010). Getting the statement of deliverables right is important at this stage, as they are the organising principle for the rest of the WBS.

Each deliverable will require a number of activities to be conducted. Activity is the next level down in the WBS, and is basically a manageable collection of related tasks that contribute to a single deliverable (Hill 2010).

Each activity in turn will require the completion of a set of tasks. These categories (tasks and activities) are highly variable depending on the needs of the project, and in some ways are defined by their relationship to one another and to the higher levels of the WBS. Thus tasks are discrete pieces of work that are needed to complete a single activity.

A **work package** includes all the scheduled activities and tasks (with milestones) that are required to complete a deliverable in a WBS (Kloppenborg 2009). A work package should be detailed enough to facilitate further planning, such as scheduling tasks and determining resources, and to assist the project manager to maintain control of time and resource use during implementation.

Constructing a WBS

The common steps are logical: start with the deliverables, break each one into meaningful activities, and then into tasks, in descending order. It is important that each element in the WBS is described clearly, but briefly.

The WBS is usually presented in a graphic format. Figure 6.1 shows a vertical WBS, with deliverables listed on the left and dropping from top to bottom. Activities are listed in a column to the right of each deliverable, and tasks follow the same format. The work represented in this way for each deliverable is sometimes called a '**deliverable leg**'. A WBS can be presented in many other formats, including horizontally (with deliverables listed on the top from left to right) and can be shown in outline only (Hill 2010).

The WBS can also be presented in project stages, or according to responsibilities (such as for different team members or groups). Display by stages is used for multistage projects, and the deliverables for each stage are grouped. Display–by–responsibilities brings together the activities for

Figure 6.1 Work breakdown structure

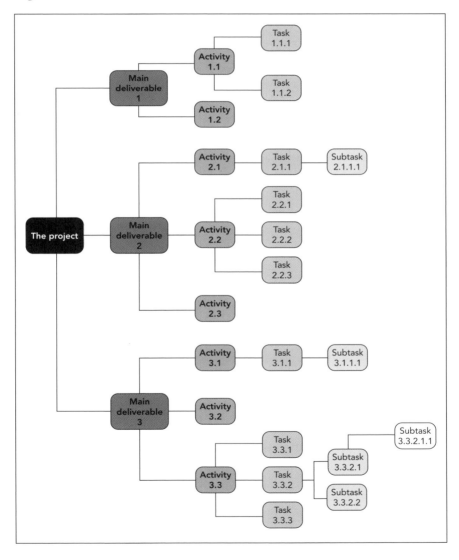

which individuals or groups (often with specific skills) are likely to be responsible. These different ways of presenting the WBS will suit the needs of different users and audiences.

Normally, two to three activities for each deliverable are enough (Hill 2010), but there are no standard rules for this—you just need to be able to visualise the sequence of events. It can be hard to know when to stop dividing activity into smaller elements. One rule of thumb is the **80 hour rule** (Kliem et al. 1997): no single activity or group of activities should require more than 80 hours (or two weeks) of work. But this rule may not always apply, depending on the nature of the project, its activities, and the skill and experience of the project team. Another way of thinking about this question is to make sure that activities are set so that they don't last longer than the time between meetings of the project board or committee. This way, regular progress reports will be clear, tracking and monitoring easier, and the team will have some achievements to report. So the best rule is the 'common sense rule'—be as detailed as makes sense to you!

We have described above the 'top-down' approach to constructing a WBS, but it can also be approached 'bottom-up'—that is, by identifying all the work elements first and then grouping them to form the higher levels (Hill 2010). In reality, the process often involves a mix of the two—as you specify activities and tasks, any omissions or errors in the way the deliverables have been described come to light, and can be corrected. The WBS in Figure 6.1 is displayed according to 'deliverables' or 'products' of the project.

The construction of a WBS and the specification of individual work packages allows time, cost, schedule and even associated risks to be estimated individually, and also enables responsibilities to be allocated to members of the project team. Figure 6.2 details one of the work packages in the WBS for a project that aims to reduce steroid use among high school students.

Estimating time and using scheduling tools

Managing time is important for projects, and estimating the time required for tasks and activities is a reliable way to establish a schedule and milestones against which progress can be assessed (Kliem et al. 1997; Martin 2002). The development of the WBS gives you a starting point for performing the next difficult task of project planning: estimating the time

Figure 6.2 Work package details

Project: Reducing steroid misuse by students in our city	Work package: Improvement of students' attitude towards their appearance		
Project aim: To reduce the prevalence of androgenic anabolic steroid misuse among grade 10 public school students in the City Council Area	Deliverables: Eighty per cent of grade 10 public school male students in the City Council Area developed a positive attitude towards their appearance		
Activities	**Resources**	**Expected duration**	**Cost**
Conduct promotional campaign	Project officer Printing services School teachers' time	2 months (85 hrs) 1 month 15 hours	
Facilitate a series of group discussions among 200 grade 10 female and male students to encourage positive and effective communications in the first 12 months	Project officer Project team leader School teachers	8 months (0.7FTE) 8 months (70 hrs) 5 months (300 hrs)	
Facilitate a series of workshops for 200 grade 10 students focusing on consolidating and advancing changes (in the second year of the project)	Project officer Project team leader School teachers	8 months (260 hrs) 8 months (85 hrs) 5 months (300 hrs)	

required to complete each task and the whole project. This is best done bottom-up—that is, by firstly estimating the time required for each task and work package (Kloppenborg 2009). In principle, the summation of the time required for the completion of all work packages gives you the estimate of time required for the completion of the project. However, not all work packages or tasks have to be completed in sequence, so the whole may be less than the sum of the parts. It is also important to remember that the three factors—time, cost and quality—must be considered together. Time estimates can't be finalised without reference to cost and quality considerations.

Our research indicates that the challenges in estimating time requirements relate to four factors. Firstly, some tasks may require specialised skills and expertise, which makes it hard for nonexperts to estimate the complexity and therefore the time required. Secondly, good estimation requires a substantial investment of time and energy, which may be exactly what is lacking. Thirdly, differences between senior management and project staff regarding expectations and quality requirements can complicate this task, as can a lack of support or involvement by management and key stakeholders in the planning process. Finally, financial constraints also challenge both the planning and execution of projects.

The time needed to complete key activities in the project is almost certainly not known in advance, so estimation is vital (Martin 2002). But estimating time and resources realistically at the beginning of a project is not easy. As one of the senior managers we interviewed observed:

> From my experience in developing budgets I think a couple of things are quite difficult and one is actually estimating the length of the project. Some tasks might take longer and a lot of times we underestimate how long it takes.
>
> *(Health senior manager)*

One of the common mistakes made during estimation is overestimating the productivity of project staff (Roberts 2011). If nonproductive time is not taken into consideration during estimation, the timescale for project completion won't be realistic. There will inevitably be tasks that are necessary but not directly related to the building blocks in the WBS. Industries other than health and community services often use a standard productivity rate of between 56 per cent and 80 per cent (Roberts 2011) to recognise these factors. On the other hand, overestimating the time needed for the completion of the project is equally undesirable. Goldratt (1994), in his study of techniques for removing unnecessary padding from the estimation of project tasks, suggested that managers tend to overestimate the time needed for individual tasks by a minimum of 100 per cent.

In the case of small projects, some form of brainstorming with colleagues may be a good approach. For large-scale and complex projects, estimates can be tested by seeking second opinions—by talking to people who are not involved in the project but have had experience in similar projects. You can also use estimates from projects that are similar to yours as a guide. For large-scale projects, trialling and revising is the key:

> Well I think it's just trial and error. I think it's based on what you know about your business; what you know you can achieve in a

certain time; what you can foresee is going to be the length but, as you say, that can always change.

(Hospital clinical leader)

Even though estimating can be hard, putting time and resources into it means you are more likely to avoid unsuccessful project implementation.

Gantt charting

The Gantt chart is one of the oldest project management tools, and one of the most commonly used methods of presenting schedule information (and of charting actual progress). A Gantt chart plots activities (in rows) against the timeline (in columns), thus showing the relationships between them. Gantt charts can also show the resources required for a particular task or activity, as well as the relationships between the tasks, milestones and baselines; and can be used to track planned and actual progress (Meredith & Mantel 2009). Figure 6.3 presents a simple Gantt chart for the project of conducting a community survey.

For a simple project a Gantt chart may be hand drawn (or word processed in a table format); for more complex projects it may be developed using a computerised tool such as Microsoft Project software. Gantt charts are useful in both the planning and implementation phases of the project because they are simple, easily understood and very effective for showing the status of a task or a group of tasks against the schedule. Their limitations include the fact that they can be difficult to update

Figure 6.3 A simple Gantt chart

	Task name	Duration	April	May	June	July
1	Literature review	20 days				
2	Conduct survey	39 days				
2.1	Prepare questionnaire	10 days				
2.2	Pilot questionnaire	7 days				
2.3	Review questionnaire	7 days				
2.4	Interviews	15 days				
7	Analyse results	15 days				
8	Write report	65 days				
8.1	Structure and outline	5 days				
8.2	First draft	27 days				
8.3	Second draft	12 days				
9	Preparation of report	0 days				18/07

if there are lots of changes and can become unmanageable in more complex projects.

The many other project management charting and scheduling techniques include network diagrams, critical path analysis (which shows the critical tasks and times for the project to meet a deadline), and the **program evaluation and review technique** (PERT: one of the first formal methods developed for scheduling projects). They are not often used in health and community services, other than in some building and IT projects, because there is not the same focus on managing technical tasks and resources concurrently. Descriptions and tips on how to use them are included in many texts.

Larger and more complex projects are often better handled in stages. This is helpful when there are major unknowns which will only be clarified as the project progresses, or when there is major risk that needs to be mitigated. For example, building and information system implementation projects are often divided into stages due to their size and complexity. Projects that aim to design and test new models of care, on the other hand, may be organised in stages because the testing process can't be determined until the design is known. Structuring projects in stages—where design/redesign in the light of learnings from the previous stage is a planned strategy—can be an essential aid to maintaining quality, momentum and control.

Some of the breaks between stages may be designated 'go/no go' points, where there is an opportunity to assess whether the project should continue, be substantially revised or abandoned. An example of a go/no go point might be the moment of sign-off following acceptance testing of software or a new laboratory method. Staging of this kind can also assist in creating a more comfortable framework for the consideration of major changes. The establishment of planned times and methods for deciding whether particular designs work, and whether the benefits and costs are in the right balance, can make it easier for decision-makers to agree to proceed with projects, even though they have misgivings about some of the possibilities or find uncertainty difficult to manage.

In order to design a project in stages, key decision points and decision-makers need to be identified very early in planning, along with specifying the criteria and information they will use. Important meetings need to be timed accordingly (while allowing for some slippage). In effect, each stage needs its own plan. While this may sound daunting, it can in fact make the task easier because the planning is broken down into manageable pieces, and detailed planning for later stages can be deferred.

Planning for human resource needs

People make projects happen.

(Verzuh 2011)

Working out the human resource requirements and how to build the project team are critical tasks for most projects, and some steps can be taken at the planning stage, based on the project charter (discussed in Chapter 5), WBS and timelines. Often writing the detailed project plan is the first task of the newly appointed project manager, so some of the key questions below may have already been answered:

- What kind of skills are needed to achieve this project?
- Are these skills available within the organisation or will they need to be sourced from outside?
- Which of those skills are needed by the manager?
- What other people with particular skills are needed, and how much of their time, how many of them?
- How will technical or specialist expertise not available among team members be brought in?
- What processes will be used for selecting the project manager and other team members?
- How much authority over team members will the manager have?

This is the stage when organisations that have nurtured project capability and skills within the organisation (or have more project experience or more internal resources) will be seeing the benefits of their investment. On the other hand, contracting for project management and team members may be a necessary or desirable strategy.

Because of the uniqueness of each project, it is rare for an organisation to have all the necessary skills in-house for a major project (Healy 1997: 15). This is as true of human services as any other area, and so consultants and temporary specialist staff are often engaged either to work directly on a project or to backfill operational positions. The nature of the relationship between contracted staff and the project manager or sponsor needs to be well planned and communicated. During the planning phase it may be useful to draft position descriptions for the project team members, which enables a quick start to the recruitment process if required.

Consultants can add real value to a project by bringing high-order skills, up-to-date knowledge, the objectivity of an outsider and a greater freedom to deliver uncomfortable messages or challenge the prevailing culture. On the negative side, working with consultants and contractors can be a knowledge drain for the organisation and may also require additional resources to manage the contract. Contracts can include a requirement for the consultants to transfer knowledge and skills, and to hand over all the 'intelligence' gathered as part of the project (in the form of briefings as well as organised files). This can ensure that the organisation gets value for money from the consultancy and will reduce the likelihood of future dependency on a particular consultant or firm.

Budgeting

A budget is a financial document that projects income and expenses. It is a written forecast or plan of what managers expect to happen in the future, quantified in terms of dollar inflows (revenue) and dollar outflows (expenses) (Van Horne 1998). Organisations use budgets as planning tools to allocate resources and to evaluate their overall operations. For a project, the budget specifies all costs involved in completing the project and the funding or revenue required to cover the costs (when revenue and costs are equal, this is a 'balanced budget'). The fundamental purpose of the budget is to enable the project manager to measure actual results against the plan (Day et al. 2004). It provides important information to guide project monitoring and control, and indicates where action is required (to reduce overall expenses, or change practice and systems to reduce supply costs, and so on). A good budget is built on good estimation of time and costs, and on consideration of uncertainties and risks, and makes adequate funds available for achievement of the project goals.

Budget development

The literature on project budget development and control (including Kovacevic et al. 2001; Dobie 2007; Kloppenborg 2009; Hill 2010; Roberts 2011) generally recommends that those preparing budgets undertake the following steps:

- Conduct a thorough analysis of the scope of work and tasks, activities and timelines, labour and other resources required to complete the work—the WBS provides a solid basis for completing this step
- Assign realistic monetary values to the required resources, based on estimates for each item—thus forming a preliminary budget
- Identify risk factors and allow for their potential impact on the budget—the risk management plan provides a good basis for calculating a contingency allowance for risk
- Present and discuss the preliminary budget with senior management (and perhaps financial sponsors if relevant) to test that your thinking and calculations are in line with expectations, to explore the reason for any differences and then resolve them.

In the implementation phase the budget becomes the primary document for monitoring and controlling costs. The budget format depends largely upon the project itself and upon organisational systems and financial management practice, but a single spreadsheet can be used to list all project revenue and **expenditure items**. Expenditure items can be grouped according to type, for example **labour** (staff) or non-labour (equipment/materials) items, fixed versus variable expenses, or initial costs versus those occurring later in the project. Budgets are normally '**cashflowed**' (that is, costs are allocated over the weeks or months of the project) so that expenditure can be monitored against time and linked to progress.

Identifying and estimating costs

If it's something new it's often difficult to work out what the cost is going to be. I suppose it's about using the information that you have got . . . there's always unknowns about what the uptake might be or something that you haven't foreseen.

(Hospital clinical leader)

Cost estimation is an unavoidable part of developing a budget. Project managers may be able to get valuable help from the organisation's finance staff, but those staff will need good instructions about what to include, and the expected size or volume of the resource (for example, programming time to capture the data from a new care process; duration of a group program; number of participants for a community activity; how many test kits for a new approach to monitoring a chronic disease; and so on). Essentially, the following resources in the project must be planned for, and their costs estimated:

- The staff (labour) required to do the work of the project, both within and outside the organisation. The time of the project manager and project team members, even if they are salaried staff, should be included, along with any additional expertise that may have to be 'purchased' in the form of legal advice, consultants, statisticians, agency staff, and so on. Check your organisation's financial policies for the need to include labour 'on-costs' (typically up to 25 per cent on top of base rate salaries, which effectively covers the costs of superannuation, workers compensation insurance, leave entitlements, penalty rates and so on.)
- Equipment, services and materials that will be needed for conducting the project—that is, the **direct costs** of setting up the project office, and all the consumables required.
- Specialised resources or products that need to be purchased as part of the deliverables (for example, hardware and software needed to implement a new patient management system, or access to a gym to trial a physical activity program for people with a disabling condition).

As far as possible, costs should be based not on 'guesstimates' but on data gathered from the organisation's finance and payroll systems, together with prices from suppliers and quotations for any externally provided services or equipment. If the project will last for more than one year, costs should be indexed for inflation or salary increases (finance staff can advise on formulae for doing this).

Again, it is sometimes difficult for one person to come up with a comprehensive list, and team brainstorming and fact-checking is often the fastest way to develop a list and estimate the cost of each of item (Kovacevic et al. 2001; Lock 2007). Detailed estimating is often one of the first tasks facing a newly appointed project manager. If a working group was formed at the project initiation phase, this group can contribute. Project managers can also seek input from others likely to be involved in the project, and from senior management and finance staff.

One of the participants we interviewed gave a good summary of the process for developing budgets for complex projects:

> For capital building projects that are large with multiple vendors, I use the following techniques: appoint an independent cost consultant to ensure independent management of the budget; develop a planning budget which is tied to the original business case; use established cost estimating techniques including 'rule of thumb'; always include contingency.
>
> *(Community manager)*

One way to check your list of expected cost items is to consider two categories: items that are unique to the project (these are more likely to be identified); and items that are necessary to the project but more routine—these are more likely to be forgotten. Table 6.1 provides a few examples using the two projects mentioned earlier in the book.

Table 6.1 Examples of project cost items

Title: Hip fracture prevention project	Title: Androgenic anabolic steroids prevention project
Cost items unique to the project • Employment of a specialist nurse • Purchase of hip protectors • Development of risk assessment manual *Cost items that may be common to all projects and easily forgotten* • Preparation for staff training • After-training follow-up • Supervision of implementation of risk management among staff • Survey on effectiveness of staff training workshop • Data collection and analysis, and report writing for the survey	*Cost items unique to the project* • Employment of a facilitator to conduct the education workshop • Development and printing of workshop materials *Cost items that may be common to all projects and easily forgotten* • Preparation of workshop • Workshop participants recruitment and selection • Pre- and post-survey on changes in knowledge and practice among participants as a result of the workshops • Data collection and analysis, and report writing for the survey

Other common cost items such as supervision of the project leader, overhead costs, publicity (for both the project and staff recruitment) and promotion may also be easily forgotten.

Participants in our research confirmed that it can be hard to estimate staffing requirements, timelines and other costs correctly. Sometimes the budgeting requirement is skipped entirely for internal projects, and those responsible simply incorporate the project costs in their ongoing operational budgets. When this works, it is simple and perhaps more comfortable, but when it doesn't—for example, by causing unexpected and unexplained cost overruns—the consequences can be troublesome for the budget holders. It is a good idea to be clear about those costs that will be absorbed in operational budgets (with the agreement of the budget holder) and those that need to be included in the project budget.

Direct and indirect costs

Expenses or costs can be categorised as direct or indirect (Martin 2002; Courtney & Briggs 2004). Direct costs are incurred by and for the project—that is, they would not be incurred by the organisation other-wise. They may include the following:

- Salaries, wages and other benefits (such as superannuation) for those working directly on the project including the project leader, project officers and others who contribute (perhaps on a part-time or sessional basis) to getting the project done
- Communication costs such as project-specific telephone charges, printing and postage (such as a community mailout or the printing of special project stationery)
- Transport and travel costs incurred by project staff specifically for project activities (such as taxis, flights or special courier services used by the project)
- Equipment and computer software or hardware used solely for the project (such as the hire of computer voting equipment for a community meeting)
- Project staff training and professional development that is neces-sary for the project
- Consumables and stationery used in project activities (such as refreshments supplied to focus groups).

Indirect costs, often called 'overheads', are incurred for a common or joint purpose and therefore cannot be identified readily and attributed to a particular project. These costs may be necessary for the implementation and completion of the project, but are shared with other activities within the organisation. Project indirect costs may include:

- salaries, wages and other benefits for staff who don't work on the project, but who administer or otherwise support the project as part of their ongoing job, such as department administrator, ward clerk or IT staff
- general purpose equipment, computers and software such as word processing programs
- space and utility costs
- general purpose office supplies such as paper, pens and toner cartridges
- routine internal courier services and general postage
- routine printing, reproduction and photocopying
- basic telephone line charges, pagers, local calls and voicemail
- subscriptions, organisational memberships, practice books, and journal and magazine subscriptions used by the organisation
- insurance such as public liability
- supervision of project leader.

In some circumstances, expenses normally charged as indirect costs may be charged to the project as direct costs. For example, large, complex projects that involve extensive data accumulation or surveying may need to employ an administration officer to support this work rather than using existing administrative staff—this would be a direct cost. Similarly, some routine costs are routinely allocated to their end use, and if the project is included in this procedure (for example, a large or externally funded project may require a cost centre in its own right) these costs will be allocated as if they were direct.

Getting the budget right: not too little, not too much

The art of budgeting is to set the costs correctly, without either 'padding' the budget through unrealistic assumptions (like zero delays in recruitment or allocation of staff) or, on the other hand, overlooking or underestimating significant cost items. Budgeting can be hard, according to those we interviewed:

> Budgeting is hard because as public servants we're not really in touch with reality when it comes to budgeting . . . It would be

helpful if we could get some benchmarks about what's a fair price for things . . . There's no guidance anywhere for that, you just have to intuitively work that out.

(Senior health manager)

Health and community services face constant pressure to reduce costs without compromising service delivery (Brown et al. 2003; Dwyer 2004). Projects are usually not immune from this pressure, so the principle of cost containment needs to be applied throughout the project planning process.

The golden rule of budgeting

The 'golden rule' for developing a good budget is to ensure all items that are included in the budget are allocable, allowable, reasonable and necessary, and are being treated consistently (Queensland Treasury 1997; Martin 2002; Dobie 2007).

A cost is *allocable* to a particular project when it can be directly attributed to it—that is, the cost really belongs to the project. For example, a project leader purchases equipment to be used for work on a funded project. The equipment is allocable to the project as a direct cost. The project leader also purchases printer toner for his office printer which is used for all of his unit activities. This is not directly attributable to any one project, and is therefore not allocable and may not be charged as a direct cost to the project. Instead, costs of using the printer for project work can be allocated to the project on the basis of either an actual usage charge (such as using a project pass code) or a rule of thumb (for example, 20 per cent of the printing for this month is for the project).

Only costs allowed by the organisation's policy, or accepted as common practice, can be included. For example, a project leader has a project officer working on the project. This is an *allowable* direct cost of the project. However, the project leader may consider discussing the project with the project officer over dinner. If meal expenses are not allowed by the organisation's policy, this is not an allowable cost and may not be built into the project budget.

A cost must be *reasonable* and *necessary* for the performance of the project. For example, a project leader purchases lab supplies to be used for the project. The supplies are reasonable and necessary for the project and may be charged to the project as direct costs. At the same time, the project leader also purchases an electron microscope on sale at a price hard to pass up. It is not needed for the current project but may be needed for an upcoming project. The microscope is not reasonable and necessary for the performance of the current project and may not be included in the budget.

Costs incurred for the same purpose in like circumstances within the organisation must be *treated consistently* as either direct or indirect costs. That is, if the organisation generally treats a particular type of cost as direct (and therefore allocable), the same cost can't be treated as indirect anywhere within the organisation. The reason for this rule is to avoid incorrect or double charging. Similarly, current practice should be used as the guide when deciding how to name and categorise each budget item, for consistency in accounting treatment.

Budget items

The project budget should be developed to include all predicted expenses that will be incurred during the whole project period—and all relevant income that will cover predicted expenses. In principle, project expenses and income should be equal, to ensure that the project can be financially self-sufficient. A budget usually includes six categories in the expense section as detailed in Table 6.2. However, the grouping of budget items can be different between organisations depending on their accounting practice. For example, budget items can also be grouped as fixed, variable and semi-fixed costs. Finance staff can be very helpful with getting the categories and grouping right. They are also more likely to support the project manager with budget problems during the project if they understand the budgeting decisions and if the budget has been correctly structured and documented.

Sources of funding and other resources

In health and community services, the resources needed for the project may be acquired from four major sources:

- External funding or material resources (such as access to meeting rooms in the local hospital for a medication management workshop being run by the community health service)
- Internal allocation of funds (such as from fee-for-service activities or interest earned)
- Internal 'in-kind' funding (for example, staff time, office space, administrative support—not cash)
- Donations.

Table 6.2 Budget categories and items

Budget categories	Items
Labour costs (staffing)	• Salaries • Consultancies • Agency costs • On-costs: superannuation, recreation leave, sick leave, possibly workers compensation insurance, allowances and so on.
Administrative costs	• Staff supervision • Financial management • Administrative support
Operational costs	• Postage • Stationery • Meeting costs (venue hire, catering, and so on) • Office space/rental • Travelling expenses • Telephone/fax/mobile/internet • Advertising and marketing costs • Printing and promotional materials • Staff training and development
Capital costs (major asset purchase)	• Equipment • Office furnishing • Office building or vehicles (very unlikely for projects) • Software • Vendor/contractor costs
Evaluation costs	• Design of data systems or questionnaires • Contract with external evaluator
Other items	Necessary items specific to the project and not included above

Source: Liang (2011)

Each funding source brings obligations and expectations, from very formal funding contract obligations to government funders, to expectations for acknowledgement and appreciation (for example, if the organisation's volunteer or fund-raising organisation funds the project).

There may also be resources that are readily accessible to the project without cost or obligation. In the case of a project aiming at improving medication management skills of people with high blood pressure, brochures may be freely available to the project from the local health department. These contributions should be included in the detailed budget on the 'revenue' side, even when the dollar value is zero. This not only makes it clear to funders that all available resources have been marshalled by the project (something they generally appreciate), but also benefits future planning for projects and ongoing services. Projects are often used to pilot new ways of providing services or managing operations, and a full record of all resources required for a successful trial provides an important input to decision-making about ongoing implementation of the project outcomes (for example, by routinely offering a new service or doing business in the new way).

Constructing a detailed budget

If a work breakdown structure has been prepared, the details of work packages provide the basis for writing a detailed budget. The activities and tasks are already specified, and it is then more straightforward to identify the resources required and estimate their costs. For example, if a nurse with expertise in high blood pressure education is needed for workshops in medication management, the first step is to find out what classification or salary level should be offered for this nurse specialist (based on education and experience requirements). The next steps will be to calculate how many days or hours of time are needed per week or per workshop for all required tasks (such as preparation of workshop materials and data recording), and for how long (how many weeks or workshops).

Once all required resources for each work package have been listed, they can be entered into the budget template. A good budget template will remind you of what may have been left out.

For a project where a WBS may not be justified, or may not yet have been completed, a good estimation of project costs can be prepared by listing all the essential tasks and the resources and time required to complete them, and then calculating their costs. There are many templates for developing a full project budget, and the organisation may well require a certain format (which can be modified if necessary for the special requirements of the project). Figure 6.4 is an example of a budget that has been developed for the androgenic anabolic steroids prevention project.

Figure 6.4 Project budget example

Resource (itemised)	Funds sought from Dept of Health		In-kind donation from CHS	
	2013	2014	2013	2014
Staffing				
Project Team Leader 0.4 FTE (Health Service Manager Award Level 2 Year 1)	$34 726	$36 115		
Project Officer 0.5 FTE (SACS Award Youth Worker C IV Year 1)	$24 164	$25 131		
School Teachers 600 hours (State School Teacher Award Step 8)			$8362	$8697
Administration Support 5 hrs/w (SACS Vic Award Class II Year 2)	$5555	$5777		
Total staff on-cost (23.5%)	$15 144	$15 759	$1965	$2043
Staff training and skills development				
Three days group facilitation training for project officer	$1155			
Half-day team building training for project manager	$275			
Drug and Alcohol Prevention Conference in Victoria registration	$715			
Administrative costs				
Project Team Supervision from Director of Young Program (5 hrs/month, $62/hr including on-cost, 4% increase for year 2)	$3762	$3913		
*Insurance & financial management	$8958	$8273		
Operational costs				
Office rental ($85/w, 4% increase for year 2)			$4420	$4597
Telephone/fax/mobile cost (2 mobile $60/m + $60/m landline)	$2160	$2246		
Printing and postage for letters to parents ($0.70 x 800 per year)	$560	$560		
Stationery and other printing ($150/m)	$1800	$1872		
Recruitment costs, e.g. project staff and facilitators	$2640			
Tea, coffee, etc. for student workshops ($8/person x 600 students x 5 sessions per year)	$24 000	$24 960		
Tea and coffee and lunch for three days intensive training for health professionals ($25/person x 3 days x 120 people)	$9000			
Venue for health professional training: $350/day x 3 days x 4 series)			$4200	
Venue for student workshops ($130 x 5 sessions x 20 series per year)			$13 000	$13 520
Travelling expenses (local travel to meetings and to schools and workshops 35 km x 164 travels x 0.62/km)	$3559	$3702		
Capital costs				
Laptop computer with software	$2300			
Desktop computer with software			$1800	
Office furnishing			$650	
Fax machines			$350	
Two telephone sets	$550			
Data projector (rental) ($437.50/w for 4 weeks in first year)	$1750			

Resource (itemised)	Funds sought from Dept of Health		In-kind donation from CHS	
	2013	2014	2013	2014
Promotional costs				
Poster and brochure design	$1375			
Printing poster ($28 x 120)	$3360			
Printing of brochures ($0.55 x 1500)	$825			
Printing of training materials for health professionals ($30 x 120)	$3600			
Printing of information for parents ($0.55 x 600)	$330	$330		
Printing of handout for students at the workshops ($3 x 600 per year)	$1800	$1800		
Evaluation costs				
**Internal evaluation cost		$7237		
External evaluation consultant ($190/hr x 76 hrs)		$14 440		
Total cost	$153 363	$152 115	$34 747	$28 857
Total cost including 10% GST	$166 788	$167 326	$38 222	$33 082
Total funds being sought from DoH	$334 114			
Total donation in-kind	$71 304			
Total budget	$405 418			

* Calculation of 5% insurance and financial management: 5% of all cost of the individual year expenses including funding being sought and donation in-kind (excluding evaluation cost)
** Calculation of 2% internal evaluation cost: 2% of all cost of all expenses for the whole project (both years) including funds being sought and donation in-kind

Source: Adapted from Liang (2011)

Budgeting for contingencies

When the budget is taking shape, it is helpful for the project manager and working group to make time to reflect on the uncertainties in the project itself that could affect the budget. The risk management plan (see Chapter 5), along with the budget document, provide the starting point. The following questions might be relevant:

- Does the budget include any identified contingency funds, or estimates that already allow for potential contingencies?
- Are there any special expectations by senior management or the funder that have cost implications?
- Is there professional expertise within the organisation that the project can utilise?
- Is there any professional expertise that is critical to the project and may be hard to find? If so, what are the implications?
- Are there any expected difficulties in recruiting staff? Can any existing staff be allocated to the project?

- Have evaluation costs (based on the evaluation plan and funder requirements) been included?

Answers to the above questions may have different but significant effects on the project budget. For example, if difficulties in staff recruitment are expected or internal recruitment of staff is impossible, staff recruitment costs need to be included in the project budget. The impact of delay in staff recruitment on the project costs should be factored in. Sometimes a potential project is just too complex to estimate with confidence— and perhaps too complex for the organisation to conduct. Flexibility in changing the shape of the project and in budget development is important:

> Instead of having a cast of thousands and changing the whole way the public system interacts with the private system we've decided just to . . . scale it right back and the result of that little bit of prep work should be the bigger project. So you just scale the project back to a level that can be easily managed.
>
> (Senior health manager)

> Sometimes funding bodies are a little bit rigid about those things and they say 'oh take the evaluation out or take it down' so what we're going to do is try and have a formula that is flexible but that has some benchmarks in it. We're not there yet; we haven't done that yet, we've just talked about it.
>
> (Community manager)

The project business case

> Sometimes it's a case of if you can show a positive business case, how cheaply can you do it and what can you get away with . . . very rarely are you in a position where you've got more money than you know what to do with.
>
> (Senior hospital manager)

In project management, a business case is essentially a project plan and financial analysis that quantifies and schedules the costs of a project as well as the benefits and direct cost savings or increased revenue arising from the project. A positive business case is one in which the benefits (which normally arise after the project is completed) outweigh the costs. The origin of the term lies in the small business field, where typically an owner of a small business (or intending owner of one) needs to present a positive business case to their bank or potential investors in order to get the capital needed to open or extend the business—that is, it is essentially a plan that demonstrates that the business is capable of repaying the investor or financier (Overton 2001). Preparing a business plan can be important for small business owners for other reasons, as it essentially forces the owner to answer the question 'how can this business be profitable?'.

The concept of a positive business case is a bit different for projects in health and community services. The question may instead be 'will this project enable us to do something differently or better without additional cost—can we make this pay for itself?' (the 'break even' argument). For private providers of services, the question may be 'can we make this pay for itself and generate at least an acceptable surplus?'.

If the costs of a project are significant and sources of funding are hard to find—but there are potential returns if the project works—a well-argued business case can give decision-makers a compelling reason to find the money and make the investment (Dobie 2007). In some situations, a signed-off business case may be required to get a mandate for the project. In addition to showing how innovative and effective the proposed inventions or initiatives could be, the business case needs to address how the proposed project can justify the resources required (or how implementation of its outcomes will be sustainable); how it will contribute to the achievement of the organisation's and/or funder's strategic goals; and, if possible, how it will complement or enhance other approved initiatives and thus maximise their benefits. However, the business case does not need to be complicated:

> We don't get right into the nitty gritty and overcomplicate it. The same with our business case, we've got a board that—I mean it's a very talented board but we provide a business case that's easy to read, easy to understand and deals with all the complex issues.
>
> *(Senior hospital manager)*

Writing a business case

The business case document will be used as a tool for raising interest among key stakeholders and potential funders. It should address the following questions:

- What strategic benefits will the project bring to the organisation?
- Why is the project good value for money, given that the organisation will make a considerable investment in the project?
- What are the consequences for the organisation if it were not to conduct this project?
- What is the evidence that supports the case (in a form that is useful for decision-makers)?
- On what criteria will success of the project (and a decision to proceed with implementation of the result) be based?

All of the detailed planning and budgeting work will provide much of the information needed for the writing of a business case. The business case should be as concise and clear as possible, while including all necessary practical details. There are plenty of business case templates available (for example: http://www.projectmanagementdocs.com/templates/business-case-template.html) and Figure 6.5 provides a generic business case template for consideration.

What about projects with no positive business case?

For some projects, there is no way that the project results can be applied without additional costs—for example, the introduction of a new keyhole surgical technique will probably expand the number of patients who can be treated and therefore cost more, even if the procedure itself is more efficient. A new diversion program for young people at risk of offending will probably bring no financial benefit or reduced costs or 'offsets' to the provider of the program. In this sort of case, the question may be 'can we justify this additional service to funders on the basis of health or welfare benefits?'. This is essentially the argument that social harms or cost will be prevented or money saved elsewhere in the health or welfare system—even if there are extra costs for the organisation that provides the service. If this is the basis on which justification will rest, an economic analysis may be what is needed (see Chapter 4). Case 6.1 illustrates this point.

Figure 6.5 Business case template

Executive summary
❏ A concise summary (ideally on two pages) of the content of the document, including all recommendations. It should read as a 'stand alone' document, and should not introduce any material not found in the body of the report.

Sign-off sheet
❏ For recording project sponsors' and proponents' signatures, committing them to act on the business case, or recording their support.

Current situation
❏ A statement of the background and current context with relevant facts and judgements backed up with evidence (expressed in numbers where possible).

Future state
❏ The intended, predicted or desired future situation or environment. That is, the realisation of goals and strategies; the future role delineation; risk profile; and service models and so on. Any assumptions should be clearly set out and supported with relevant data or other evidence.

Policy issues
❏ The broad policy, political, legislative and organisational constraints within which the business case must fit. For example, government policies, social justice considerations, legislative requirements, accreditation.

Strategic alignment
❏ Alignment of this initiative with organisational/government strategic goals.

Gap/needs analysis
❏ A statement of the problems, gaps or needs that the project seeks to address, supported with relevant data and analysis.

Options for action
❏ All feasible options to address the problems or gaps within the policy constraints. Each option, including the 'base case' or 'do nothing' option, should be described in enough detail to establish workable alternative courses of action. Each option must be capable of standing alone.

Analysis of options
❏ Qualitative and quantitative analysis including income and expenditure streams; sources of funds for capital and recurrent costs; economic analyses (such as cost utility); risk analysis; volume of outputs or services; strategic considerations; and timing. The analysis of each facet should conclude with a definitive result or solution, since these results will be used for comparison and selection of a preferred option.

Evaluation and selection of preferred option
❏ Based on the results of the steps above and a clear statement of the criteria and process, the preferred option is identified (and usually also appears in the executive summary).

Recommendations
❏ The preferred option is presented in the form of a decision or action for decision-makers to endorse or decline. Any needed information about decision-making and approval processes and the management of perceptions should be included.

Implementation plan
❏ Specifies the team or individual responsible for implementation, and outlines the main components of the project plan.

Appendices (if needed)
❏ Material referred to but not included in the business case. For example, members of the project team; additional financial or service data and analysis; demographic/population profiles; equipment lists; and references.

Case 6.1 Positive health outcomes: negative business case

A children's hospital identified that many young parents were unaware of the dangers of shaking their babies (in a misguided effort to make them stop crying). Using donated funds, the hospital undertook a major education campaign for parents using educational videos and other resources. After a year the hospital was able to demonstrate a dramatic reduction in the incidence of shaking and in the admission of babies with the resulting brain injuries. Because of technical aspects of the hospital's funding, revenue was potentially reduced rather than enhanced by this outcome. No positive business case for this intervention could be presented, but the merit of the project is obvious.

Summary

- The work breakdown structure (WBS) is useful for estimating the time and resources required for the project.
- WBS enables sequencing of project tasks, and estimation of their duration. It also allows the identification of time and resource issues in the project planning phase.
- Estimation of time and costs is important to good project planning. However, estimation is never perfect for something that has never been done before. A number of strategies can be adopted to improve the quality of estimation.
- A budget is an important document to plan income and expenses for the project, and provides project managers with the ability to measure actual results against planned expectations.
- Budgets should be based on experience, good understanding of the project and its tasks, and team effort. Budget development should be guided by the important features of costs—budget items should be allocable, allowable, reasonable and necessary, and be treated consistently.

- A business case can assist in clarifying the importance or priority of a proposed project, and will help decision-makers to understand the value of the project, leading to their support.

Readings and resources

Hill, G. M. (2010). *The complete project management methodology and toolkit*. Roca Raton: CRC Press.

Courtney, M., & Briggs, D. (2004). *Health care financial management*. Sydney: Elsevier.

Roberts, P. (2011). *Effective project management: identify and manage risk plan and budget keep project under control*. London: Kogan Page.

Project Management Docs, 'Project business case template': http://www.project managementdocs.com/templates/business-case-template.html

'Project budget templates', Australian Centre for International Agricultural Research: http://aciar.gov.au/ProjectTemplates

7

The implementation phase: getting it done

Control and monitoring during implementation
    Keeping to the plan
    Controlling project scope—change control
    Controlling the project schedule
    Controlling the budget and resources
    Managing quality
    Managing risk and contingency
    Managing evaluation
    Status reporting
When things go wrong: getting back in control
Summary
Readings and resources

The implementation (or execution) phase is the moment when the rubber hits the road for the project—when the long-planned actions are taken, and strategies are implemented. When the project is underway the project manager's focus shifts to two key goals: making the project happen, and monitoring and measuring progress to ensure that the project stays on track.

In this chapter, we first discuss the management and leadership tasks of this phase, and the challenges of achieving change in the project, including some brief outlines of theories about change. We suggest some methods for making sustainable change happen, and for dealing with the project politics and resistance to change. The final section of the chapter addresses tasks, tools and techniques for controlling and measuring the project's progress to successful completion, including status reporting.

Getting started

> Where you 'walk the walk' as the project manager
> *(mastering-project-management.com)*

Implementation of a project is about leading and motivating people, and coordinating human and other resources to carry out the plan. Controlling a project is about ensuring that its objectives are met by monitoring and measuring progress regularly to identify variances from the plan—and taking corrective action when it is needed (PMI 2008).

The Project Management Institute (PMI 2008: 55–64) describes the process involved in the execution of a project as:

- project plan execution—performing the activities on the plan
- quality assurance—making sure the overall performance of the project meets relevant quality standards
- team development—developing individual and group skills/ competencies to enhance project performance
- communication and information distribution—making needed information available to project stakeholders in a timely manner.

We would like to add to this list:

- Stakeholder management—working with stakeholders as the project unfolds, shoring up their commitment, responding to their concerns and monitoring any shifting alliances.

The sum total of these activities can be overwhelming for the project manager. So where do you start? The project plan is the key, and this is when the benefits of planning are realised. Sometimes the first activity is a project launch or kick-off meeting with the steering committee and the project team, which marks the commencement of the project proper and can help the team to bond and focus.

Where the project manager has been appointed after the development of the plan, a review of the plan and any associated business case is a good place to start. Is the plan realistic? Are there any glaring omissions? Was some of the planning not detailed enough? Have project activities commenced already? If there are problems with the plan at the commencement of the project implementation, now is the time to address them—the sooner the better.

For the project manager new to the project and/or the organisation or unit in which the project sits, the first step is to understand the project's history and the context. Finding out the background to the project, how it developed and who was involved can assist further on if the project seems to hit brick walls, is being 'white anted', or when something is happening that you just cannot put your finger on.

As the project is getting started, it's often a good idea to think about the sticking points that are likely to arise and how they could be resolved. This requires careful listening, honest thinking and informed logical analysis. It can be helpful to stand back from daily concerns and really analyse what's going on around the project and where the problems are likely to come from. One method is to tell yourself the story of how this project succeeds: what are the key mysteries that are solved, the lucky breaks, the turning points that will make the difference? This technique can be used to identify the negatives as well: if this project were to fail, what would the causes be, who would be the villains of the story? These techniques are a kind of rehearsal for managing and leading the project, and can be used in preparation for important presentations or meetings as well.

Leadership, motivation and teamwork

> Project implementation is primarily about people. Only people can produce work and effort so your first concern must be how to lead and motivate your team.
>
> *(Webster 1999: 117)*

Leadership, particularly for motivation and good teamwork (working together to a common purpose or shared goal) is essential in creating successful project outcomes. The guidelines in the following list can help project managers to achieve these objectives:

- Do not lose sight of the goal of the project—whatever strategies you develop, they must be focused on achieving this goal
- Timelines are important—while some flexibility might be necessary, too much flexibility will see you lose control of the project
- Problems and potential problems must be identified and dealt with—they will not go away, and might get bigger and come back to bite you at the most inconvenient time
- Attention to detail is essential—it can help you identify problems and keep your eye on emerging issues, so keep good notes and records
- Keep your eye on the ball—work the project; it will not happen by itself
- Walk your talk—make sure that you do what you say you will do; model good project management practice
- Hone your communication skills—be a good listener and approachable; provide clear, easy-to-read written reports and memos that are short and to the point
- Improve your facilitation skills, especially in meetings—make all meetings productive or people will stop attending

- Recognise the skills and work of others, give praise where appropriate—give credit where credit is due, but also deal with non-performance
- Take responsibility—beware of blaming others for problems
- Encourage good working relationships—through good humour, a positive attitude and a 'we can do this' approach
- Aim to be someone who creates and gives out good energy—rather than a black hole that sucks the energy out of others.

Action learning

One of the more challenging leadership tasks is ensuring that the project team 'rolls with the punches' and is constantly assessing and refining the evolving project's methods and focus. Action learning (or the related idea of reflexive practice) is an approach that may be useful for this task. Action learning is the practice of thoughtful consideration (and discussion) of events, a process by which people make sense of their experience and its meaning (Revans 1998; DeFilippi 2001; Leggat et al. 2011).

Project managers can promote action learning in their teams by the simple method of encouraging thoughtful discussion and analysis of any aspect of a project that seems either troublesome or potentially rewarding, or that might be seen as a 'critical incident' (for example, a walkout by a stakeholder). Regular team meetings can be used both to address normal project business and to encourage reflection and learning. The major challenge with this technique is to establish an environment of trust and safety so that team members can engage in open, thoughtful discussion; and then to maintain a climate of safety through mutual commitment to confidentiality and constructive use of discussion outcomes. At the commencement of the project and when the team is established, it may be useful to conduct a project induction and orientation process where the project 'code of conduct' can be discussed.

Establishing the project team

Recruiting a project team can be a challenging and fraught process, undertaken in what is often the rush to commence the implementation phase of the project. Determining who will be part of the team happens during the initiation and planning phases, and the recruitment process may be formal or informal. It will depend partly on whether recruitment is internal or external. If external, the formal recruitment process will include advertising, shortlisting, interviews, letter of offer and contract; or engaging with a contractor to provide specified services. The process may be informal when organisational 'rules' allow and leaders prefer.

Internal recruitment involves the secondment of staff to the project team. This may be a formal process of advertising project positions internally, then interviewing, followed by selection and appointment; or people may be identified and approached by the project sponsor or manager—some negotiation with their usual line manager may be needed. Internal recruitment can be a sensitive and emotionally charged process, with line managers sometimes perceiving that they are losing quality staff to the project with negative effect on their department. The availability of funding to support backfill, to enable the staff member's normal work to continue, can also be a critical consideration. It is important to be flexible, communicate well and negotiate with managers regarding the terms of the secondment, lead times, commencement dates and duration, availability of backfill funding, dual reporting and how the process of transition at both ends of the project will work.

Tips for effective project team recruitment:

- Develop position descriptions for each project team role and ensure that the sponsor or steering committee approve them.
- Open recruitment processes (including advertising the project team positions and conducting interviews) are generally more effective both for getting the best people and for satisfying general staff perceptions of fairness and opportunity.
- Involve the key stakeholders and clarify your authority in the decision-making regarding project team appointments.
- Clarify expectations regarding formality of recruitment processes required for your project from an organisational, human resources and industrial relations perspective.
- Communicate effectively and often with all the stakeholders, in particular the managers to whom the staff report.
- Be familiar with the policies and processes for effectively transitioning staff onto the project team, including employee contracts, variation of employment forms, timesheets, rostering systems, budgeting and cost centre management.

Managing project staff

Building a project team that works well together is a key part of project success. All the normal requirements of good people management and effective teamwork apply. Good management of a project team also requires effective responses to three important issues:

- The problem of two bosses
- The challenge of rapid skills development
- The question of retention of a temporary team until their work is really done.

Some team members will probably only report to the project manager for the duration of the project, or may continue to be supervised by their normal line manager throughout. Openness between the two managers involved can help avoid a situation where the team member feels pulled in two directions. A clear delineation of the split in reporting relationships is essential. For example: Who approves leave? Who does performance appraisal? Who can make demands on the person's time and for what? How will the managers keep each other informed in a way that is fair to the staff member?

In many cases, team members may have only some of the skills the project needs. Although the project cannot wait for long-term skill development, all team members need to be confident in the specific methods and tools that will be used in this project. It is therefore usually a good idea to hold training workshop/s for the team to explain and finalise the project's chosen methods, tools, templates and reports, and to train team members in their use. Topics such as running effective meetings, process mapping techniques and interviewing skills could also be covered. Competence can improve rapidly when some training (and opportunity to ask questions) is provided; when tools and templates are used consistently across the team; and when team members are able to use the project manager and other leaders as models. Staff should be given the opportunity to identify their areas of interest and strength as well as those areas where they lack skills or confidence. Then either their roles can be structured accordingly, or further skills training can be arranged.

Finally, towards the end of the project, there can be a tendency for team members (and maybe the manager) to focus on returning to their units or seeking further project opportunities, rather than on finishing the project. It is a good idea to raise this issue at the beginning and work out strategies for meeting both the needs of the team members and the needs of the project.

At the least, the manager, and maybe one or two others, could be contracted until well after the expected completion date to allow for slippage and for project closing and bedding-down activities. This will give them a period after the project is practically completed to focus on their next moves. Team members and the project manager could also negotiate agreements with the operational manager to cover problems with timing or any other aspect of the return to the operational area and agree on a process to be followed if these contingencies arise.

Early attention to these important issues, and establishing an environment of safety and clear expectations among the project team, will pay off in enhanced capacity to deliver results—and to weather storms—as the project progresses.

Problem-solving skills

During the course of the project it might become obvious that the project team has gaps in its skills and knowledge, or conflicts might emerge between team members or other groups and individuals. This can be one of the most challenging things that a manager has to deal with, inside or outside a project. While there are many techniques and methods for dealing with conflict, basic problem-solving skills are particularly relevant.

It is important to keep an open mind in order to recognise problems as they begin to emerge in the project team. Webster (1999) suggests the following problem-solving process:

- Accept that a problem exists and resolve to take action
- Dispassionately gather the facts
- Define the problem
- Understand what is causing the problem
- Engage the team in contributing to both understanding the problem and finding solutions
- Plan the response and implement it.

The 'GRPI' framework (goals, roles, processes and interpersonals) is an effective tool both for promoting good teamwork and for analysing and addressing team problems (Johnson 2010). It is sometimes drawn as an inverted pyramid, to make it clear that shared goals are the starting point (the biggest element) for good teams. The other elements are clearly defined roles for team members (no gaps or unhelpful overlaps); reliable processes and systems (that enable people to get their jobs done); and, only then, interpersonal factors. That is, poor team functioning may appear to be caused by interpersonal problems, and is often where the pain is felt, but the source of the problem probably lies elsewhere, and the manager needs to pay attention to factors higher up the order. Figure 7.1 illustrates this model.

Figure 7.1 The GRPI framework

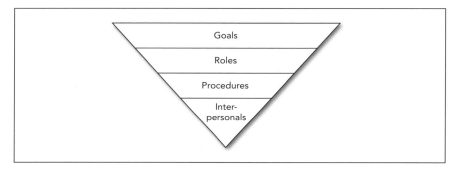

Conducting effective meetings

Project meetings fulfil many important functions in most projects, and are necessary for effective communication. They will be more effective if they are properly scheduled, have a well-structured agenda, and are briefly recorded in minutes that include required action and reporting. There will be different types of meetings with different people participating—project team, steering committee, executive briefings, stakeholder meetings—which will probably require various approaches to decision-making, structuring the agenda, facilitating discussion and reporting progress and outcomes.

Good meeting and facilitation skills can help to save time, diffuse conflict and make things happen. There are two underlying principles in facilitation. The first is the need to be efficient: people are busy and hate to waste valuable time in unproductive meetings. The second is participation: people need to have their voices heard and feel that they are contributing if they are to have some ownership of the project and maintain their commitment. We suggest the following guidelines for good facilitation:

- Always have an agenda—no matter how small and informal the meeting

- Know the meeting timelines and stick to them—start on time (latecomers will probably get the message), put time limits against agenda items and stick to them unless there is a very good reason not to
- The facilitator does not have to know the answer to every question—put difficult points back to the meeting or agree how they will be 'parked' and dealt with later
- Keep things moving along—do not let participants ramble
- Encourage some people to speak
- Be prepared to shut others up—nicely!
- Keep on track—don't be taken off into irrelevant issues
- Look for answers to difficult problems
- Make sure every issue has an action—even if it is just 'defer to next meeting'
- Make sure each action has an owner who is responsible for making it happen
- Keep notes or minutes
- Make sure you revisit minutes at the next meeting and deal with any matters arising
- Keep a record of attendance.

Achieving sustainable change

We turn now to the major implementation challenge the project team will face—achieving change through the project. Projects can be the biggest single enablers of changing the way organisations do things, by bringing the right people together to work towards project goals.

Usually the whole purpose of a project is to bring in something new or to do something differently—that is, to innovate. Innovation is defined as the successful implementation of something new or, more simply, as 'putting ideas to work' (Department of Industry, Science and Resources 2000: 9). In health and community services, as in other spheres, innovation happens when a new process or system is introduced, even if the agency is not the first in the world to undertake that particular change.

In this section we focus on projects that need to achieve sustainable change in some aspect of the existing work system, power structure, working relationships, roles or responsibilities of people and teams— that is, where the change will affect people and their work. A lot has been written about achieving change in organisations, and much of it applies to projects. We briefly review some of the major theories and approaches to change that are relevant to project management and the politics of change, and then address the ways people respond to change with particular reference to the central theme of resistance.

Most of the early research in this area focused on the technical aspects of project management and the successful management of individual projects (Partington 1996). It presented a rational approach to change in project management processes, emphasising the importance of goals, planning, tasks, staff, tools, timelines and resources but ignoring the people side of change. Yet our research and the literature (for example, Andersen et al. 2006) indicates that it is the people side of project management, more than any other single factor, that leads to project failure.

Participative approaches to implementing change

The organisational change theorists tell us that while directive processes can achieve change quickly, it is the more participative approaches to change that create a sense of ownership and involvement among the major players (Dunphy & Stace 2001). For example, research from the UK, Australia and New Zealand (Perkins et al. 1997) demonstrates that senior medical staff are more likely to support change when they have had some involvement in the decision-making processes. The main critiques of such participative change processes as 'organisational development' are the slow pace of change—which is achieved in small, incremental steps—failure to deal with the difficulties of participation, and lack of acknowledgement of issues of power.

The change that is part of the project is by its very nature proactive change, although the project may have originated as a response to an external event or crisis. Projects are also generally aimed at sustainable change—that is, making sure that something not only changes in the short term but also becomes embedded in organisational practice. Both these characteristics tend to argue for a well-structured participative approach.

McElroy (1996) articulates a clear argument in favour of the use of projects for achieving organisational change. He contrasts four methods of implementing change:

- Education and communication—persuading staff of the need
- Participation—staff assist management to define the change and the change process

- Intervention—management defines the required outcomes but uses projects to enable participation in the process
- Edict—where management gives precise instructions to be followed.

He concludes that intervention is the most effective. In this method, leaders make strategic decisions and set the parameters, using project methods to engage affected staff in designing and implementing operational change accordingly. The project approach is recommended because it enables the setting of clear goals and scope—ensures they are authorised before the project begins. That is, management (in signing off on the project charter and plan) accepts its responsibility to resolve the question of 'should we seriously try this?' up front, before the work commences. While there are no guarantees, this method helps project teams and sponsors to handle the natural resistance from those who are affected, and to hold stakeholders to the project mandate.

One of the problems in health and community services is that much of the change that has taken place in the past has been radical, top–down, directive change, as organisations have had to respond quickly to budget cuts, policy directives and shifting government priorities. Strategies that Kotter and Schlesinger (1979) describe as manipulation, co-option, and explicit and implicit coercion have been used to implement change. But, as many managers have found, there are problems with these strategies in the human services industry, and in any case they are most often not available to project managers. Case 7.1 covers some other approaches to change.

Managing participation

We advocate the use of participatory methods to engage staff and stakeholders and enhance the momentum of the project. But there is also 'tyranny of participation' or 'death by process' to consider: endless meetings, surveys, workshops and interim reports that waste time, cause the project to lose momentum and reduce good will. The challenge is to balance openness, transparency and consultation with maintaining momentum and sticking to the project's goals and scope.

There are two main levels to managing participation. One is the project's leadership structure, including the engagement of stakeholders in committees (discussed briefly in Chapter 5 and addressed later in this chapter). The second is broader participation by staff generally and by members of stakeholder groups. The key to success with these

Case 7.1 Change makers: the surgeon, the scientist, the nurse and the administrator

There are many approaches to change not recommended in the management literature. These are some that can be observed on field trips:

- The surgeon: Make the decision and do it. Just do it. (The crash or crash through approach.)
- The scientist: Get the right answer. Verify the data and the logic. Then it will just happen—won't it?
- The nurse: Look over there! See, it didn't hurt a bit, did it? (The distraction method.)
- The administrator: Process, process, process. (Change by exhaustion.)

Each of these can work for some things, sometimes. But there are better ways.

methods is structured participation, with well-designed processes that ask the right questions at the right stage, and recognise that people want to have their say but are also busy.

The most effective participation processes use a range of methods tailored to the needs of the project, the participants and the style of the organisation. They pose questions for debate and solution, relevant to the participants, that will be genuinely useful to the project, and are held at the right time in the project's life. They make the givens explicit, such as decisions already made by the executive or board, or the implications of government policy or legislation, to provide a framework around the areas of discretion. And they do not ask people to start with a blank canvas if this is not the real situation.

For some people, being able to make a submission is important. Alternatively, when the project team needs to understand the thinking of particular groups, confidential one-to-one or small group discussions with project staff, or others who are trusted by the group, might be the only effective method. This approach can enable the project team to get the insights it needs and lets the relevant group see that their views are taken seriously. Safeguards to protect the rights and interests of line managers can be built into this process, so that it doesn't become either a witch-hunt or a method of undermining the effectiveness of management.

For some questions, straw polls using computer-based 'voting' on questions (or its low-technology equivalents like post-its or dots on wall posters) can produce surprising results that capture the majority view more accurately than open discussion, which may be dominated by vocal and higher-status individuals. Computer-based voting systems have the advantage of allowing instant collation of results and producing graphs that clearly demonstrate the balance of views. Alternatively, sometimes a conflicted group will agree that the project should consult an independent expert and will accept that person's opinion on particular issues.

The general principle is to use appropriate methods to gather meaningful results with an explicit method of analysing and using the outcomes. Most importantly, there needs to be a method of closing off the participation exercise and moving on. For further information about how to manage participation, skilled workshop facilitators are recommended.

The politics of change: managing the shadow side

In any discussion of organisational change, the issues raised are often essentially 'political'. By political we mean the methods by which people seek, acquire and use power (Pinto 2000: 85). This brings in the power structure and relationships, and the tactics and strategies people use to enhance their power or their access to prized resources. It also includes the alliances and groupings that share and use power and influence, and the resources, information and support on which they are built.

One of the reasons that many change processes fail is that the proponents do not understand the politics of change. The health and community services sector is comprised of many powerful stakeholders who do not always have the same interests and often compete with each other for power and prestige. Organisations survive in an environment of contradiction and conflict. They must manage tensions between providing a service and balancing a budget, between their espoused policy and their actual practice, between centralism and localism, between professionals and managers, and between change and tradition and comfort.

Managing change is a political process, and some writers argue that the ability to achieve change is a function of power and influence rather than method (Stephenson 1985). For Nadler and Tushman (1997), change management is a problem of power, of anxiety and of organisation control. They believe the response should be focused on shaping political behaviour, motivating constructive behaviour and managing the transition.

While some elements of the power structure (such as formal hierarchies, controls and resource allocation) are overt, much of the politics of the organisation, and of the project, happens in what Egan (1994) calls the 'shadow side'. According to Egan (1994: 41) the shadow side is:

> all the important activities and arrangements that do not get identified, discussed, and managed in decision-making forums that can make a difference. The shadow side deals with the covert, the undiscussed, the undiscussable and the unmentionable. It includes arrangements not found in organisational manuals and company documents or on organisational charts.

The shadow side is outside ordinary managerial intervention and can substantially affect productivity and the quality of working life, both positively and negatively. A supportive organisational culture is a powerful positive element of the shadow side. Other positive aspects include informal advocacy on behalf of the organisation, which many staff undertake both within and outside of work settings, and informal networks of communication that flow under and around formal channels and help both managers and staff know what is going on.

Negative elements can include things like:
- entrenched enmity between functional managers (affecting the ability of their departments to work together)
- a culture that accepts poor performance by favoured individuals
- executive or board members influenced in their decision–making by loyalty to an outside force (such as their professional association or their family's interests) rather than the organisation
- approvals processes that are not understood and documented
- manipulation of meeting agendas and minutes (matters not discussed at all, or discussion not minuted accurately).

There will always be a shadow side, and organisations will always have politics. The question is not whether, but to what extent and in what directions (helpful or harmful) do organisational politics operate? Good management, tolerance of difference and debate, and open communication will tend to minimise the space that the shadow side has to work in. That is, bringing important issues into the open and dealing with them in a careful way will reduce the need for negative shadow-side activity. Projects can be an opportunity to shine the spotlight on forgotten cupboards and remote attics in the organisation and to deal constructively with shadow-side issues (but judgement is needed to decide which doors to open when).

There are many managers, and project managers, who feel that politics is a dirty business and would prefer to operate above or outside it. Politics can indeed be unpleasant, but staying outside it is really not possible. Dealing ethically with organisational politics, and your own role within them, requires skill and strategy. The first skill is the ability to see and 'read' what is going on. The second is to know how to challenge the negatives creatively. The third is to be able to turn discomfort and disruption into learning.

Project managers by and large do not have a strong or stable power base (Pinto 2000), and learn to cultivate influence instead. The need for influence is made stronger by the fact that projects often exist outside the formal structures and so all resources must be negotiated and bargained for. Lack of authority—for example, to conduct a performance review of project team members—also limits power, and project managers may even be managing their peers or their superiors. They have little managerial control in this situation and so human skills become very important. As Pinto (2000: 86) argues, 'successful project managers are those who intuitively understand that their job consists of more than simply being technically and managerially competent'.

This has many implications for project politics. The first is that project managers must understand and acknowledge the political nature of most organisations, especially the influence of key stakeholders. The second is that project managers must learn to cultivate 'appropriate' political tactics.

One important tactic is to use the 'WIIFM'—what's in it for me?— principle. For example, departmental or unit loyalties and interests are usually more immediate and more powerful for most people than commitment to organisation-wide concerns, especially in large organisations. It can therefore be helpful to analyse proposals and issues in the project from the point of view of each of the departments or groups whose contribution, or acquiescence, is needed. When people respond to a proposal by asking 'what's in it for me?' they are offering the project manager an opportunity to explain why they should support the project.

Alternatively, power can be enhanced through tactics that level the playing field. In health and community services, knowledge and expertise are highly valued, and project leaders who hold or develop a superior knowledge base, and use it to add value for the stakeholders, can enhance their power base and thus be more effective in negotiations (Pinto 2000).

Stephenson (1985) argues that the necessary skills include negotiating and bargaining, urging and cajoling, and coping with resistance. He also suggests assessing the power of opposing forces, forming coalitions and choosing optimal timing for action. In real life, the champions of change juggle opportunities, problems, the shadow side of the organisation and their upward management issues—and a combination of good luck, good ideas and good management gets them through. Whatever model or strategy for change management is used, the 'pointy end' of change management in projects is dealing with the response typically labelled 'resistance'. We use this label in the following sections, but it's important to note that some of what is called resistance to change is motivated by concern about technical errors or wrong-headed policies. A lot of this concern can be met with a listening ear, and improvements to project design can result. Not all resistance is motivated by self-interest, nor is it necessarily a threat to the project.

The rationale of resistance

When changes are proposed, the people who will be affected begin calculating gains and losses in relation to two basic questions: 'What's in it for me?' and 'Will it really happen?' (Skinner & Price 1990). There are some good reasons for the tendency to resist change. Those who are comfortable with the ways things are will often see, perhaps correctly, that they have something to lose, including some of the power or influence they currently hold. And they will often have some power which they can use in order to resist, as Case 7.2 illustrates.

On the other hand, those who stand to gain from a proposed change, either personally or because they agree with the goals of the change, are

Case 7.2 Understanding resistance to change

The consulting doctors whose lives are organised within a complex web of sessional arrangements and a daily round of attendances at several hospitals have good practical reasons to resist a proposal for daily morning ward rounds in one of the hospitals in which they work. And the reasons persist even if payment for their time is adequate, and regardless of how much more efficient it might make the care of their patients in that hospital. They also have the power of their independence, and often that of the market (in other words, they will be hard to replace). Gnashing of managerial teeth, and exhortations to 'think of the greater good', are unlikely to be very persuasive. For change to happen, the consultants' real difficulties and best interests are going to have to be understood and responded to, as the power of the manager to force change is probably limited.

in a position of uncertainty. Their active support generally depends not only on whether they can see that there is something in it for them, but also on whether they believe it will really happen.

Resistance can occur anywhere. Individuals and groups without strong power find ways to resist change, and senior managers whose areas are affected by the project might also use tactics of resistance. Some of the direct and indirect approaches to the art of resistance are summarised below (with apologies to the animal world).

The White Ant: Sneaks around pointing out all the possible downsides, no matter how farfetched or unlikely. Undermines and actively works against change. 'If you go to daylight saving, the cream will curdle, the scones won't rise and the curtains will fade.'

The Beaver: Mobilises resentment about every problem, and every change in living memory, to build a dam of resistance. 'You could let them know how angry you are about the new intake process by helping me to stop them from changing the team structure, and anyway we haven't recovered from the rostering system they put in three years ago.'

The Tortoise: Never comes to meetings about proposals s/he doesn't like the sound of, and doesn't read emails advising how to contribute; moves slowly on everything related to the proposal, and grumbles quietly in the tearoom about not being consulted. 'Don't talk to me, don't change anything without talking to me, and don't move so fast.'

The Kangaroo: Usually a senior manager, hops from one idea to the next, and appears just before sunset wanting to change the project scope. 'You've built a great battleship, now let's make it fly.'

The Red Herring: Finds a very interesting distraction to complicate and bedevil the path of the project. 'The new system will be great, but only if we can reorganise the Christmas holiday roster by Friday.'

The Worry Warthog: Has a negative disposition and has ten reasons why nothing can be done and change cannot be introduced. 'If you change the process, the sky will fall in and there will be mass walkouts of all the staff.'

Changing resistance

Perhaps one of the most famous models of change is Lewin's force field analysis. Lewin (1958) sees the change process as a struggle between the driving forces for change and the restraining forces for maintaining the status quo, as represented in Figure 7.2.

Figure 7.2 Force field analysis

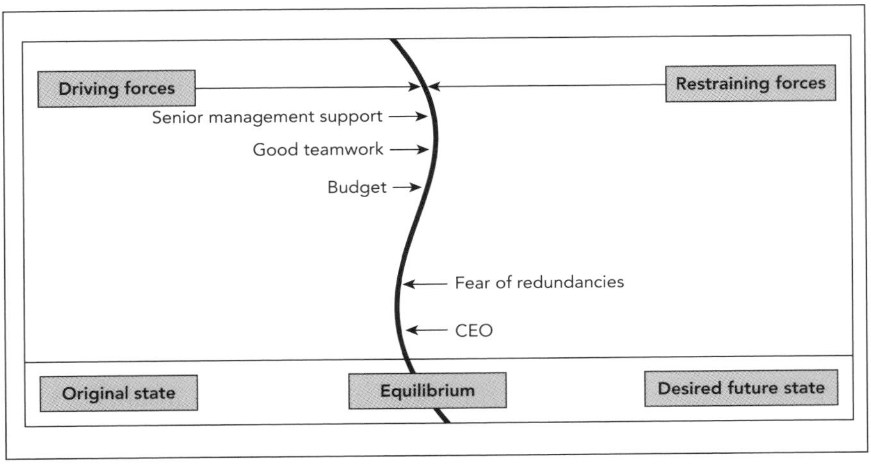

Source: Adapted from Martin and Henderson (2001)

According to Lewin's model, the change agent should first of all identify through qualitative research the forces for and the forces against the change. An assessment can then be made as to which of the forces is strongest and weakest, and what strategies are needed to support the positives and weaken the negatives. In Figure 7.2, the project is championed by a senior manager, and supported by an effective, confident team (which needs to be sustained through the change process) and a budget imperative. The change could affect staffing numbers, so fear of redundancies is a force of resistance. The senior manager also knows that although the CEO professes support, she will be watching to ensure that the senior manager is kept in line. The senior manager believes this problem can be headed off, so the CEO is therefore listed as a weak force of resistance.

Martin and Henderson (2001) also point out that 'pull' tactics as well as 'push' can be used to move the line of resistance: sometimes it is more effective to focus on weakening resistance rather than on strengthening the forces for change. For example, the fear of redundancies will not go away because positive forces are strengthened. It is more effectively dealt with directly, by providing cast-iron assurances (if there really will be no redundancies) or by negotiating principles to protect the interests of staff (if redundancies are on the cards). On the other hand, the weak potential for problems with the CEO is best dealt with indirectly through strengthening the positives of trust and accountability in the manager's relationship with the CEO.

The next stage is to unfreeze patterns of behaviour on the individual level, the level of structures and systems, and the organisational climate/interpersonal level—that is, to make the behaviour patterns less stable, more questionable and more open to change. This is followed by the stage of movement or transition, followed by the refreezing of the new patterns of behaviour or the institutionalisation of change. Lewin recognised that the intervening transition requires careful management and thoughtful implementation tactics.

The value of Lewin's model is that it can be applied to almost any change situation. It provides a way of identifying the hidden forces that can derail the change process and the analytical basis for a strategy for dealing with them. Like the stakeholder analysis map in Chapter 5 (Figure 5.1), it can help the project manager to identify the important resisters who need to be removed, and the important supporters who need to be nurtured and mobilised. One of our research participants agreed that dealing with resistance is central to the project management role:

> It's identifying obstruction and dealing with that early and having an idea of how you're going to deal with that obstruction and at the same time having the commitment from the key people that you need.
>
> *(Hospital senior manager)*

As noted above, there are always good reasons for resistance. Tactics for reducing or removing resistance are generally based on an understanding of the needs and interests of the groups involved. For project managers who lack coercive power there are two basic routes: buy them off or change their hearts and minds, or both. It may be possible, for example, to move the positions of some of the players on the field so that interests are realigned, or to convince them that change is needed through well-presented data and analysis. For some people, being brought into the tent (that is, included on committees or in formal and informal meetings) will be enough to move them from mild resistance to open-minded monitoring or even a position of support.

Listening to resistance

> Strategically, we should belittle our enemies, but technically, we should take them very seriously.
>
> *(Mao Zedong)*

There is temptation for the project manager and team to label resistance as a bad thing and to reject it. However, it is likely that at least some of the resistance will be well informed and well intentioned, and potentially valuable for the project. Understanding and analysing the sources of resistance will often lead to change in the project—for example, staff members' concern about the costs of change may be based on a more detailed understanding of current reality than the project manager enjoys. Each issue must be judged objectively on its merits and project managers need to challenge their own assumptions. There is usually great value in meeting with stakeholders who are resisting change or opposed to the project. Only when you meet face to face can you understand the stakeholder perspective (and assumptions) and genuinely work towards resolving identified issues, as illustrated by Case 7.3.

Resistance to change is not always a bad thing, as Kahn (1982: 416) argues:

> In considering obstacles to change, we must keep in mind the deceptive nature of our concepts. When we want change, we speak of those who do not as presenting obstacles and resistance. When we want stability, we speak of perseverance and commitment among those who share our views. The behaviour of people in the two situations may be identical; it is their stance relative to our own that dictates our choice of language.

When project changes are made in response to feedback from stakeholders, the situation should be presented openly and with appreciation. It is the project manager's responsibility to follow through with any needed adjustments to the project plan, including its timetable or strategies.

Case 7.3 'I'm not using that system'

The project was midway through implementing the clinical system that included electronic prescribing of outpatient medications. Dr Smith, the head of the infectious diseases unit, had so far not accepted any invitations to join the project clinical advisory group, attend system demonstrations or provide any direct feedback to the project team. Word on the grapevine was that Dr Smith had announced her intentions at the hospital's grand round to boycott the new system on the basis that it was a 'bad system' that had failed when implemented at other hospitals.

The project manager initiated a meeting with Dr Smith to understand the issues and perceptions about the system, but also to invite her to participate more actively in the project.

The project manager soon found that both his team and Dr Smith had made some incorrect assumptions. Firstly, Dr Smith had not received the invitations to participate in the project as they had been sent to an old email address. Secondly, Dr Smith clarified that while she had had numerous conversations with colleagues about her concerns about the system, she had not announced her intention to boycott it.

Dr Smith's concerns were about the usability of the system (she had heard reports from another hospital that the system had caused complete chaos in Outpatients) and that using the system to prescribe would take too long, causing increased patient waiting times. She had also been wrongly advised that the prescribing system would not cater for the antibiotic authorisation process.

The project manager then welcomed Dr Smith's input to the project and reiterated the invitation to become involved. The project manager clarified that the team had contacted the other hospital using the system, and that the major issues causing the delay had been related to the location of the prescription printers and the old PCs that they had been using.

The project manager suggested that his team work with Dr Smith and her junior doctors to ensure that the system met the needs for infectious diseases prescribing and that the new workflow was optimised. Dr Smith went on to be one of the system's most outspoken advocates.

Case 7.3 illustrates the critical role of communication in both preventing and managing resistance. This is confirmed by recent studies which found that 'rich project communications' are a strong factor in project success (Andersen et al. 2006; Chen 2011). Participants in our research also focused on the importance of communication:

You've really got to keep communicating with people so they understand what it is you're doing and why you're doing it, so really involving people, listening to them, understanding what their issues are.

(Hospital clinical leader)

Project bureaucracy and organisational change: a paradox

We have argued throughout the book that project management is all about change. But there are two paradoxes that should be noted. The first is that an overbureaucratic model of project management might actually impede organisational change (Partington 1996). Emphasis on rigid control through adherence to detailed plans and budgets and tight timelines can work against the emerging iterative nature of many change projects in health and community services. The real solutions to problems in models of care or support systems are often not known at the beginning of a project, which may be why a project approach to the problem has been chosen. In this case, the project team and the stakeholders need to be flexible in their expectations of exactly what will emerge at the other end, how and when. The project plan is still a vital component, but the need to plan for variation is also strong. Project managers must avoid falling in love with their plans and tools.

The second paradox is the fact that senior managers may, in effect, be asked to disempower themselves and at the same impose more discipline on themselves (Partington 1996). While the organisational change literature argues that support of top management is essential if change is to be realised, in practice there is tension between project-based authority (held by the project manager) and the functional authority of line managers. As Partington notes, 'it is natural for managers at every level to struggle against the abandonment of hierarchies' (1996: 18).

Projects may also effectively ask managers to exercise their authority differently, and with more discipline. By locking managers as well as staff into specified goals, strategies, deliverables and budgets, projects can be seen as a temporary and partial stay on the ability of senior managers to change their minds and manage discrete parts of their operations separately and incrementally. In some cases, the leadership level may not have project expertise, and may lack the skills to operate competently in a project environment—for example, not knowing how to respond to the challenges of managing a matrix or juggling both projects and line operations (Partington 1996).

The solution to this second problem is a long-term one that must be tackled by the organisation as a whole. However, the project manager who is aware of these issues can at least understand some of the sources of resistance from above, and at best can design ways of working around them.

Control and monitoring during implementation

So far, we have discussed the challenges of making change happen. In the rest of this chapter we turn to some of the tools and techniques that assist project managers to maintain **control** and **monitor** the progress of projects through to successful completion. The separation between these goals is a little artificial: control and monitoring play a key role in making the project happen; and the effectiveness of implementation can either support or challenge control and effective monitoring. Some organisations have mandated methods that they use for control and monitoring of projects, and in others there is flexibility about mixing and matching tools according to the needs of the project.

Methods and tools are important for control and monitoring, and decisions should be made as early as possible about which ones will be used. You may need to import or develop your own templates, forms, and data collection and reporting processes. The challenge might be the adaptation of tools and methods to the more difficult realm of organisational change projects. We discuss several of the available methods in the rest of the chapter.

Webster (1999) suggests that three types of information are required to control a project—historical, present (diagnostic) and future (prognostic)—and that information for a good control system should be visible, accurate, reliable, valid, timely and prognostic. The project plan provides the basis for determining what information about the project's progress or performance needs to be collected, monitored and reported during the life of the project. The plan will normally cover all the project parameters that require monitoring, and hence enable the design of a monitoring system. The evaluation plan will also highlight the required areas of focus for data collection and analysis. Although exactly what needs to be monitored relies heavily on the nature of the project, it is likely that data on expenditure (compared to budget), task/activity completion (compared to the schedule) and performance (compared to the specifications) will be monitored. Meredith and Mantel (2009) suggest that while it is easy to focus on monitoring data that are easily gathered, monitoring should concentrate primarily on measuring important facets of output (for example, the extent to which system design has been completed), rather than on intensity of activity (for example, the number of meetings that have been held) (Meredith & Mantel 2009: 444–49).

There are several aspects of any project that will be challenging to monitor and control. We briefly address controlling the scope and schedule, the budget and resources, project quality, risk and contingencies, before turning to the challenge of managing projects when they get into trouble.

Keeping to the plan

Having seen that the project is well planned and scoped, the project manager must then ensure that the project progresses as smoothly as possible according to the project plan (unless variations are agreed). The amount and quality of project planning will quickly become evident in the implementation phase. Any deficiency in planning may not be the project manager's doing, as not all project managers have the benefit of being involved in the project from the beginning—but the project manager is the one who will deal with the consequences.

The tasks of planning, monitoring and controlling are cyclical. That is, the cycle of planning, checking on progress, comparing progress to the plan and taking corrective action if progress does not match the plan is followed by another round of planning to incorporate any necessary changes (Meredith & Mantel 2009: 436).

The general methods for monitoring adherence to plans are status collection and assessment against the baseline provided by the plan, and perhaps by other sources. These methods involve collecting defined information to measure the progress of both the entire project and the activities within it (Kliem et al. 1997: 202). The multitude of ways of gathering data and information on what is actually happening in the project range from the 'corridor chat' to the reports generated by an information system (for example, a financial report showing actual costs versus the budget). When the data generated are meaningful and reasonably accurate, the information can be a powerful impetus towards goal attainment—achieving milestones and outcomes—for teams and stakeholders.

Controlling project scope—change control

> Change is a healthy part of project life, but it needs to be controlled.
>
> *(Healy 1997: 256)*

During the implementation phase in any project, changes to the plan (or 'variances' or 'variations') are normal and to be expected. If there are significant variances (and they jeopardise the project objectives), the plan can be adjusted by repeating the relevant planning process—for example, reestimating the staffing levels. It is inevitable that as soon as the project plan and scope have been written and signed off, changes will occur. The important issue for control is to ensure that variances are documented, the plan is adjusted accordingly, and the variance is formally accepted by the authorised group or individual.

The scope that was planned for and agreed to in the planning phase and documented in the project plan may be challenged or may require modification for legitimate reasons. There could be a change to the contract, the deliverables, the target implementation group, the budget and the schedule, to name but a few. For example, during an information system implementation there may be a need to include further functionality in order for the system to work; or the timing for a go-live might need to be extended to ensure that all the defects and issues are fixed. However, 'scope creep' (unmanaged expansion of the project's scope) is a common and serious threat, leading to cost blow-outs, missed deadlines and unmet expectations.

The tools to manage and control project scope include:
- a change request process, most commonly using a change request form (see Figure 7.3)
- a change log that records all requests for change and their approval details (see Chapter 5)
- a process for the assessing the project impact of the change request
- formal review and approval of change requests by the steering committee, which then gives the authority to the project manager to revise the project accordingly.

Figure 7.3 Change request template

1. Project information			
Submission date:		Reference:	
Initiating party:			
Project description:			

2. Change scope	
Description of change required:	
Justification:	

3. Project impacts	
Schedule/time:	
Cost:	
Other:	
Priority:	
On approval by all parties, the required change/s will be subject to quotation/confirmation of cost	

4. Project status and currency	
Implementation details:	
Current phase:	
Implementation completion date:	

5. Approvals and signatures				
Project manager:		Approved	Yes/No	Date:
Project sponsor:		Approved	Yes/No	Date:

When the project is being conducted by external consultants, the contract will usually include a provision for variations. This protects the consultant from escalating costs due either to fickle decision-making by the client or to genuine contingencies arising in the project, things not reasonably foreseen. The contract will also usually contain clauses that enable the client to extract additional work if the variation is of the consultant's making (for example, poor modelling) or to reduce or withhold payments if the quality standards are not met.

Controlling the project schedule

The chart or graphical display is the most common and simplest way to represent data in order to monitor and control a project. A bar or line graph can easily show progress in each aspect of a project compared with the project plan. Virtually any aspect of a project can be measured, and the priority is to chart the critical factors for project success. Examples of the items that are often charted in this way include:

- project task progress (percentage completion of project tasks as a whole by week)
- staff utilisation (for example, percentage usage by week)
- performance (for example, number and magnitude of variations)
- task hours and percentage complete
- customer satisfaction measures or milestones.

For projects that are structured in stages, the finishing of one stage, sign-off and commencement of the next is another opportunity for controlling the scope and schedule. At the commencement of the new stage, progress and the potential for variations can be reviewed, as demonstrated in Figure 7.4.

Controlling the budget and resources

The budgeting and estimation of project costs is difficult and often poorly done, which can mean in turn that it is difficult to control the costs of a project against the plan. Also, if the budget is not altered when the scope of a project changes, there is little chance that the costs will match it.

Monitoring of actual and forecast expenditure against budget is probably one of the most familiar control tools in the management toolkit. Good information is an important aid to the control of costs, but in the end hard decisions may be required. There are several kinds of contingency response that might be called on—finding other sources

Figure 7.4 Developing online learning modules

% Work complete	Task name	Duration	Start	Finish
100%	⊞ Concept phase	17 days	Mon 4/06/12	Tue 26/06/12
100%	⊞ Planning phase	21 days	Tue 26/06/12	Tue 24/07/12
0%	⊟ Implementation phase	36 days	Wed 25/07/12	Wed 12/09/12
0%	⊟ Stage 1 eLearning modules	19 days	Wed 25/07/12	Mon 20/08/12
100%	Drafting of eLearning modules 1–3	5 days	Wed 25/07/12	Tue 31/07/12
100%	Development of eLearning modules 1–3	5 days	Wed 1/08/12	Tue 7/08/12
0%	Testing of Stage 1 modules	3 days	Wed 8/08/12	Fri 10/08/12
0%	Communication to students	1 day	Mon 13/08/2	Mon 13/08/12
0%	Stage 1 modules go-live	1 day	Mon 13/08/12	Mon 13/08/12
0%	Evaluation of modules by user survey	5 days	Tue 14/08/12	Mon 20/08/12
0%	Sign-off Stage 1 modules	0 days	Mon 20/08/12	Mon 20/08/12
0%	⊟ Stage 2 eLearnng modules	17 days	Tue 21/08/12	Wed 12/09/12
0%	Drafting of eLearning modules 4–8	4 days	Tue 21/08/12	Fri 24/08/12
0%	Development of Stage 2 modules	4 days	Mon 27/08/12	Thu 30/08/12
0%	Testing of Stage 2 modules	2 days	Fri 31/08/12	Mon 3/09/12
0%	Communication to students	1 day	Tue 4/09/12	Tue 4/09/12
0%	Stage 2 modules go-live	1 day	Wed 5/09/12	Wed 5/09/12
0%	Evaluation of modules by user survey	5 days	Thu 6/09/12	Wed 12/09/12
0%	Sign-off Stage 2 modules	0 days	Wed 12/09/12	Wed 12/09/12
0%	Project close	2 days	Thu 13/09/12	Fri 14/09/12

of funding, reducing the scope, taking up the slack in one part of the project to support another part's shortfall, or moving team members around to meet priority needs.

Managing quality

Quality and safety are vital in health and community services, and this applies to projects as much as to ongoing service delivery. There is often a short chain between a project and the direct implications for the care and safety of patients or clients, but even when that link is indirect, the quality and reliability of the project's work and outcomes are important.

When projects are in the implementation phase, the pressure to cut corners in order to maintain progress may be significant. If performance criteria have been defined in the planning phase (see the quality planning section of Chapter 5), the focus during implementation is firstly to ensure that they are made explicit and understood by all stakeholders. This is one of the reasons why it is a good idea to set up quality assurance mechanisms that are transparent and require reporting to the sponsor or project steering committee on a regular basis.

The second focus of quality monitoring is to ensure that any variation from the quality plan is logged, documented and resolved at a high level. A procedure for acceptance of variations for the quality plan (change requests) should be formalised (usually through the project steering committee, or the customer or sponsor).

Some project teams appoint a 'quality partner': a friendly expert adviser/auditor who takes a watching brief, not waiting for the documentation of problems, but working confidentially with the team to prevent them. An experienced project manager or a person with expertise in quality in the relevant area could play this role.

Managing risk and contingency

During the implementation phase, the risk plan and the risk register (a log of project risk events) should be regularly reviewed and updated, with existing risks reviewed and reassessed, and newly identified risks added. High and major risks should be reported to the sponsor or project steering committee via the agreed reporting processes (see Figure 7.5, the project status report template) and if risk events occur, they should be reported immediately and the planned response initiated. For major risks, this will almost certainly require 'escalating' the problem to the required level of organisational authority.

Managing evaluation

The project plan should include a statement about how the project will be evaluated: what are the criteria for judging success, on what data or evidence will that assessment be made, and how will they be collected and analysed? (See Chapter 5 on planning for evaluation.)

The evaluation plan may also call for periodic assessment of the effectiveness of the processes the project uses—for example, the extent to which stakeholders are engaged in and supportive of the project. Progressive evaluation and reporting of evaluation findings according to project stages or milestones may be needed, as not all deliverables require that you wait to the end of the project to evaluate them. Reporting periodically on interim project successes may also assist with creating momentum for the project, informing later project stages and strengthening stakeholder support.

The collection of process evaluation data need not be intrusive (or worse, destabilising). Minutes of meetings and attendance records, as well as qualitative assessment by the team, sponsor and perhaps quality partner, can be used to garner information—as can indicators such as levels of attendance at meetings and capacity of the committee to make decisions in a timely way.

The work of implementing the evaluation plan should be built in as much as possible to the project's routine record-keeping and processes, so that the needed information and evidence on which a summative assessment can be made is available when the project is at completion.

Status reporting

The purpose of a status report is to advise the steering committee, project sponsor and other stakeholders whether the project is on track to deliver the planned outcomes, and to highlight where their decision-making or direct help is needed. Regular status reports help to ensure that the team has a clear view of the true state of the project, and they also mean that management stays properly informed about project progress, difficulties and issues by periodically getting the right kinds of information from the project manager. Frequent communication of project status and issues is a vital part of effective project risk management. A status report can be a formal document that is presented at meetings, or it can be a regular email or verbal update to key stakeholders.

Status reporting can commence as early in the project as required—for example, in the concept or planning phase—and early reporting can assist in both directing focus to the project and managing risk. The frequency of status reporting will vary depending on the size of the project and the requirements of the steering committee or project sponsor. It is possible to provide too much detail in status reports, which can overwhelm busy project stakeholders—the net effect being that they do not read the report or know what to action. It is important to identify and define the indicators the project is using (for example, green, amber or red 'traffic lights') to enable stakeholders to quickly understand the status of the project.

There are many status report templates available on the internet (for example, at www.projectconnections.com), and your organisation may already have a template in use. It is also a good idea to check with the project sponsor and the steering committee on their requirements for status reporting, as they may prefer the information presented in a particular way. The template shown in Figure 7.5 outlines the information that is commonly documented in a project status report.

When things go wrong: getting back in control

If there is going to be trouble in a project, it tends to rise to the surface during the implementation phase. Sometimes the problems relate directly back to the project design and plan. Perhaps the stakeholder issues are not resolvable, or the decision to proceed in the first place was not a wise one, or the political environment in the organisation is not supportive. No matter what the causes of the trouble, the project manager is the one whose job it is to sort it out. Often, the ability of the project manager to handle unexpected crises and deviations from the plan is the determining factor in whether a project is successful or succumbs to the problems that arise during its life.

So when is a project in trouble? The project's monitoring and control activities should provide the project manager with the information required to know its status, and its progress towards objectives at regular intervals. The earlier that signs of trouble are detected the more effectively they can be dealt with. One effective way of avoiding nasty surprises is to have regular reporting both from and to the project team, the steering committee or other stakeholder groups, and the customer or sponsor.

The concrete nature of the project plan (or contract) is intended as a discipline for the sponsor or the client as well as for the team. For internal projects, the project plan or the charter can act like a contract, and assist the team to resist unnecessary or harmful 'good ideas' from above.

If problems are emerging, interactions with the project team, the sponsor and stakeholders will contain warning signs that the project manager needs to assess and respond to. Examples of warning signs that may jeopardise a project include:

- essential support systems are not working or are significantly behind schedule
- senior management is not delivering on promised interventions (such as mandating requirements for staff to participate in training in new systems or procedures)
- the project itself is falling behind schedule to a point where agreed project deliverables will not be met
- essential resources (such as provision of IT services) are not forthcoming

Figure 7.5 Project status report template

Project status report for period ending: / /

1. Project summary

Project name	
Sponsor	
Approved budget	
Actual start date	
Forecast end date	
Project manager	
Current phase	*i.e. initiation, planning, implementation, closure, review*
Current status	*Green, amber or red**

* Indicator definitions: Green = [as planned], Amber = [signs of trouble], Red = [in trouble]

2. Progress

Project phases and activities	% Complete	Planned start date	Actual start date	Planned end date	Actual end date

Key accomplishments last period:

Upcoming tasks for this period:

3. Project financials <Financial year>

Cost item	Approved budget $	Actual $	Forecast overrun $	Comment

4. Key project issues

Issue no.	Issue	Management

5. Key project risks

Risk no.	Risk	Mitigation

6. Change requests

Change request	Change description	Impact

7. Key communications/Planned events

Date	Description

- stakeholders fail to turn up to important meetings
- a key quality indicator is not met (for example, a failed software test)
- the sponsor or key members of the steering committee are not attending meetings or are unavailable
- the need for the project outcome is fading because of external changes, or it is losing internal priority
- the project team is dysfunctional
- a key person is lost to the project
- the project objectives are looking unachievable—the outcome will not be sustainable (or profitable) or the service or product will not work well enough.

If signs like these are emerging, decisive action is probably required. Escalating the issue—taking it higher in the organisation—should not be seen by the project manager as a failure, given that many issues arising during the life of the project will be beyond their control. An escalation process and criteria may be defined in the project plan, and can be as informal as calling the project sponsor to brief them and request advice, or be dealt with more formally at a steering committee meeting. In some cases there will be a need to rethink and either change the project or close it down. In other cases the project manager will need to pull out all stops and 'press on' through a tight spot.

The best outcome for a troubled project may in fact be to terminate it before further investments are made or additional costs are incurred (for example, through industrial action, which damages good relations between management and staff). We discuss early closure of a project in Chapter 8.

Most successful project managers have war stories about projects that succeeded only after great adversity. Sometimes adversity is a necessary struggle to resolve an unknown factor or an error in the project design, and in the end it improves the project—though it may also add to the project manager's grey hair.

Summary

- The implementation phase is where the planned project actions are taken and strategies implemented.
- Project management is a set of methods, but it is also an art that requires flexibility and persistence. Generic project management

skills are important to the success of a project, but familiarity with the content of the project and the culture of the organisation is an advantage.

- Both technical project management skills and people skills are required by a good project manager.
- Leadership, motivation and teamwork are essential in creating successful project outcomes, and project managers need team-building skills and the ability to run effective meetings, as well as problem-solving skills.
- Projects are powerful enablers of change, and organisational change theorists suggest that participative approaches to change are likely to be more effective and sustainable than top-down approaches. Senior management needs to set the parameters and explain the 'givens'.
- Managing change is a political process and while some elements of the power structure are overt, many are embedded in the shadow side of the organisation and outside ordinary managerial intervention. Projects can provide an opportunity to bring important issues into the open and deal constructively with the shadow side.
- Project managers must listen to and understand the dynamics of resistance to change, paying particular heed to the forces for and against change, and stakeholder groups.
- Controlling project scope and managing project variance is a key activity during the implementation phase.
- Control and monitoring of the progress of project activities (according to the plan) is a key activity in the implementation phase, and there are various methods and tools available to do this. The aspects that are monitored during the implementation phase include project scope, schedule, budgets, resources, quality (or performance), risk and contingency.
- Implementation includes enacting the evaluation plan and collecting and analysing the required data. Evaluation may be conducted and reported periodically throughout the project if required.
- During implementation the project manager will be required to regularly report on the status and progress of the project.

- The project manager might see warning signs of trouble for the project, and may need to escalate or take these issues higher in the organisation in order to resolve them.

Readings and resources

Project implementation: http://www.mastering-project-management.com/project-plan-execution.html

Turner, J. R. (2007). *Gower handbook of project management* (4th edn). Burlington: Gower Publishing Limited.

Change management resources: http://www.change-management.com/tutorial-defining-change-management.htm

Johnstone, P. L., Dwyer, J. and Lloyd, P. (2006), 'Leading and Managing Change', in Harris, M. ed. *Health Services Management*, 2nd Edition, Elsevier, Sydney.

Participation resource: http://kids.nsw.gov.au/uploads/documents/tps_resources.pdf

Status report template and guide: http://www.egovernment.tas.gov.au/_data/assets/word_doc/0007/77902/Project_status_report_template_and_guide.dot

Status report templates: http://www.projectconnections.com/knowhow/subsets/status-reports.html

8

The closing phase: handover, outcomes and evaluation

Chapter outline

When is a project finished?
   Acceptance and handover
When projects fail or need to be terminated
Evaluating the project
   Learning from the project experience
   Evaluating achievement of project goals—and benefits
   beyond the project
The final report
   Presentation and handover of the final report
Sustaining project outcomes
Conclusion
Summary
Readings and resources

Sooner or later all projects come to an end. For some, closure comes with a sense of celebration and achievement. For others, closure takes place prematurely in an atmosphere of high drama, anger and blame. Projects can also drift along aimlessly until they are quietly killed off behind the scenes when no-one is looking. Sometimes projects that have been applauded on completion are found to be wanting when their outcomes are evaluated. Conversely, projects that appear to have failed can prove their worth at a much later stage. For projects that set up and trial a new service or process, there is always the question of sustainability: will it continue when the project is finally over and there is no project manager in the driving seat?

In this chapter we explore the final phase of the project life cycle: completion and closure, evaluation, and the question of sustainability of project outcomes. First of all we focus on the practical tasks of project completion, followed by a discussion of the dilemmas involved in the premature closure of projects. We then turn to the evaluation process and suggest simple practical ways to answer the question 'was this worthwhile and what have we learnt?'. We also explain more formal approaches to capturing information about the processes, outputs and outcomes of the project. The question of longer term outcomes and their sustainability is then addressed. Finally, we discuss the project report and the sharing of results.

When is a project finished?

The operational definition of project success, like the project itself, is unique. While the generic 'iron triangle' of cost, time and specifications is a useful reference point, real projects have more flavour and texture, as well as outcomes that go beyond the project deliverables. As discussed in Chapter 1, and confirmed in a recent literature review (Mortesa & Kamyar 2009), time, cost and specifications are not necessarily the main criteria in use, and stakeholders tend to assess success based on their interests and perspectives. Mortesa and Kamyar's survey results indicate that 'top management support' (usually cited as something you need for success) is a dominant *measure* of success (that is, the project is a success if the leaders believe it to be so). Whatever the complexities of defining success for each project, it is important that success is acknowledged.

When a project has run its course, the process of completing and closing it (sometimes called 'close-out') is an important final step. Unless the close of a project is actively managed, there can be a tendency for it to drift on, never quite seeming to end. The criteria for project completion are defined (explicitly or implicitly) in the project plan, typically as the finishing of all tasks in the plan, and the achievement of planned outcomes and deliverables. The final tasks could include completing training programs (and the handover of training manuals), the installation and commissioning of equipment, or the completion of operating manuals.

The key issue is to recognise and move towards a definitive end point, and then tackle the business of completion. The nature of these tasks and their timing will vary, but they fall into three main categories: acceptance and handover (the practical completion), completing the evaluation and the final report. If a project is to be quietly buried, the completion tasks are somewhat different (see later in this chapter).

Acceptance and handover

Acceptance and handover is the process of presenting deliverables to the project sponsor (or the steering committee or the person/team who will take over responsibility for the ongoing operation of the project outcomes) and getting sign-off or formal acceptance. This process also includes completing all necessary documentation and leaving project files in good order (including proper storage of data collected by the project), winding up the project team and the office, and celebrating success.

Acceptance of the project outcomes or deliverables by the authorised person or group is a key milestone. The team might be handing over an agreed new model of care, a working information system, a new policy and program for staff development, a new method of managing supplies, or a new health or social program. Practical handover of a working or satisfactory outcome should be formalised, even for the smallest and simplest projects. Recognition of the work, and clarity about acceptance (including any residual issues), are important for all who have contributed and for those who will work with the project's outcomes.

A final meeting with the steering committee and/or the project sponsor is a common method for acceptance and handover. Such a meeting can also deal with tying up any loose ends. The project might have brought into focus issues that are outside its scope to resolve and which need to be handed over—for example, participants in community consultations may have identified concerns unrelated to the project which require a response by the agency. There might also be a need to ensure that responsibility for ongoing implementation of the project's outcomes is allocated, and that tasks such as communication about the project while the new process or product is being bedded down are also covered.

There may be aspects of the project's deliverables that cannot be wrapped up at the time of completion. A key piece of equipment or software needed for the full operation of a new service might not yet be available, or the industrial implications of a change might have to be sorted out in a different timeframe from that which was possible in the project. These issues need to be clearly identified, a process for resolving them agreed, and interim arrangements to work around the outstanding issues made.

A debriefing process—that is, an opportunity for people to discuss their experiences and impressions of the project—can be rewarding in itself, and can also provide input to the evaluation and the final report. Members of the steering committee and other key stakeholders, as well as the team, might appreciate both formal and informal opportunities to reflect and debrief.

The team also needs to wind up, even if some members will go on together to work on another project or become part of the ongoing operating team. The project office may need to be closed, and its equipment distributed to the appropriate areas. Individuals sometimes need assistance in the transition back to their old jobs, or in moving on to new ones. Recognition of the transition, and practical assistance, can make it easier. Preparations for this process made in the early stages, and good management of team members, will pay off at this point.

Finally, there is a need for celebration. A special edition of the agency's newsletter, recording and celebrating the project's outcomes, might be released. A formal handover meeting might be followed by a party. The 'go-live' point for a new system delivered by the project can also be the occasion for celebration. The effort and commitment, as well as the achievements, of those who have contributed to a successful outcome need to be recognised. Celebrations of success can be a good way of building or maintaining a positive climate, and can consolidate the pride and satisfaction people feel in their work and their organisation. Parties can also be important when the news is not good, as Case 8.1 shows.

Case 8.1 Recognising handover in an outsourcing project

The hotel services staff (cleaners, caterers, porters and couriers) of a large health agency had struggled against outsourcing, and had put up an in-house bid (a proposal to keep the service in-house on new terms) which had failed. Most of them had been offered jobs by the successful bidder, but there was a lot of sadness and some anger—particularly for the long-serving staff, some of whom had been with the organisation from its beginning, and felt that they had always done a good job.

Care had been taken throughout the project to offer support to the staff, to keep them regularly informed of progress, to facilitate access to independent financial advice, to maximise their opportunities for ongoing employment and to assist those who missed out. The human resources department argued that this approach should be sustained to the end, and that there should be a farewell party for all the staff, whether they were leaving or transferring to the new employer. The general manager agreed, but approached the occasion with dread.

The usual form was to be followed—food and drink, gifts—and a short speech was definitely part of the agenda. With his heart in his mouth, the GM spoke of the good work and loyalty of the staff, as well as acknowledging that the policy requiring competitive tendering of support services was deeply unpopular and that the staff had been through a time of uncertainty and anxiety about their futures. He finished by expressing the good wishes of the hospital community. The applause was muted, and the mood sombre, but it was clear that the staff appreciated this proper farewell with the usual courtesies extended. This formal, respectful recognition of the moment of transition may also have contributed to good working relationships under the new contract.

When projects fail or need to be terminated

In our research, participants usually attributed failure to inadequacies in the planning, prioritising and resourcing of projects. There was a particular focus on factors such as failure to define the goals and scope well enough, with the result that the project goes 'off track' and is then hard to stop:

Well, you can't just keep going along . . . you limp on for three months at the end [until] you might as well say 'you know what, let's stop'.

(Government project director)

The reasons for project failure are in many ways the mirror image of the predictors of success. For example, the UK National Audit Office (Parliamentary Office of Science and Technology, 2003: 8), following a review of IT projects in the public sector, listed these factors:

- Lack of a clear link between the project and the organisation's key strategic priorities, including agreed measures of success
- Lack of clear ownership and leadership by senior management and/or ministers
- Lack of effective engagement with stakeholders
- Lack of skills or a proven approach to project management and risk management
- Lack of understanding of, and contact with, the supply industry at senior levels in the organisation
- Evaluation of proposals was driven by initial price rather than long-term value for money (especially securing delivery of business benefits)
- Too little attention given to breaking development and implementation into manageable steps
- Inadequate resources and skills for delivery of all the required outcomes.

If a project hasn't succeeded, or is limping along without a clear path to completion, the best course of action may be to abandon or discontinue it. Projects can fail in many ways, ranging from escalation ('just one more extra mile to go') through to seismic shifts in the environment. For example, in a time of national health reform, restructuring of the public health system may mean that many innovation projects are halted or abandoned because of the disruption to teams, plans and decision-making and/or the departure of project champions. When the barriers are insurmountable, or when rescue efforts have failed, the only alternative may be to terminate the project, discontinue the work and reassign the people who were working on it.

Closing a project can also be a planned contingency—for example, when the findings in one stage of a project indicate a fatal flaw in its design or feasibility and the decision not to proceed with further stages is the only option. Some of the more common reasons projects conclude prematurely are:

- loss of interest and support from management or the intended users of the project
- changing client requirements, workforce pressures, community needs or market conditions
- indecisiveness, lack of cooperation or strong resistance from important stakeholders
- change in the project itself, so that it is no longer able to achieve its original goals
- chaos and discord from an ineffective project manager or team conflict
- failure of the project outcome—that is, the product did not work, or proved unprofitable. (Kliem et al. 1997; Lientz & Rea 1998)

Terminating a project prior to its planned conclusion is difficult, because it usually involves the curtailing of a previously held vision, the breaking up of a 'project family' and perhaps the admission of failure. Termination of a project may simply mean that a project no longer continues in its current form. Meredith and Mantel (2009: 552–54) examined the varieties of project termination, calling them extinction, addition, integration and starvation. *Extinction* means the project is stopped (whether successful or unsuccessful). *Addition* means that the project is incorporated into ongoing operations as a distinct unit or department in the organisation. *Integration* is where the project disappears but elements of it are distributed within the organisation, and *starvation* is where the project still exists but budget cuts mean that no progress is achieved. An example of a project made extinct is illustrated in Case 8.2.

Sometimes commitment to a project means that efforts to revive and sustain it continue well beyond reasonable limits. In a major study of escalation (ever-expanding duration and cost) in IT projects, Keil et al. (2000) surveyed 2500 information systems audit and control professionals. The reported rate of escalation in IT projects was 30 to 40 per cent, and once escalation started, ultimate success was much less likely. Keil et al. also investigated the reasons for persistence with failing projects, and found that 'completion effect' provided the best explanation. That is, projects are more likely to continue when those making decisions

Case 8.2 Project cancelled

The project manager identified warning signs in the early days of a project that aimed to upgrade an existing intensive care unit (ICU) information system. Though the system was well out of date (about three major versions behind), and the software vendor had advised that they no longer supported the old version, the new ICU management team had shown little interest in an upgrade project. The medical director (the project sponsor) escalated the risk regarding the critical software being unsupported, and requested that the IT project manager work with the ICU staff to develop the business case for a system upgrade.

In drafting the business case, the project manager discovered that there was little support for the existing ICU system, with ICU management actively investigating systems to replace it. They felt that upgrading the current system was a waste of time, effort and money.

The project manager completed and submitted the business case (with the information that ICU had provided), but also advised that there had been lack of stakeholder buy-in. The project sponsor agreed that a new system was desirable, but believed that there was not enough money, and informed the ICU staff that the upgrade of the current system was going ahead.

The project was therefore put in motion with the business case signed off, software vendor engaged and planning workshops held. It was not until the project team was being established, with the secondment of ICU staff, that ICU management moved from passive to active resistance. One after another, the ICU manager assigned people to the project who were variously not interested, had little knowledge of the current system or were paid significantly more than was estimated in the business case. Then there was the issue of releasing them from the ICU roster, which involved a delay of up to six weeks.

The CEO was concerned about resulting variations to the project plan and timelines, and lobbying by ICU management further destabilised support for the project. The straw that broke the camel's back was a forecast overrun on the budget. The chief finance officer stepped in and announced that the project would be cancelled forthwith. The project manager disbanded the team and thanked them all for their efforts.

believe that they are so close to completion that persistence is justified regardless of additional cost. The implication is that once an IT project begins seriously to fail, it is probably best to let it go.

In health and community services, it may be that passion as well as 'completion effect' influence poor decision-making when projects are in trouble. We have already highlighted the issue of commitment to a worthy goal in the absence of feasible means, as well as the problem of conflicting goals and incentives. These factors can make success unlikely and at the same time make it easier not to manage termination actively. Sometimes, the result is that projects are left to stagnate—neither progressing towards their initial goals and objectives nor moving towards closure.

Termination is not necessarily the same thing as failure, but poor management of the process can make things worse. While it is never easy, once the decision is made it should be done quickly to minimise further waste of resources and disruption to the organisation. It is almost always a good idea to develop and articulate a clear statement of reasons for termination, and proactively communicate this message to all concerned, without delay and as consistently as possible. This tactic will not stop rumours, but it will at least ensure that they are not circulated in a vacuum. The rights and interests of the staff involved need to be protected with clear and prompt action.

One exit method for a project that is limping to a dead end is simply to declare it finished: adopt a modified goal and cut the losses, with as much dignity as possible. Recommendations for follow-up activity might be made, and evaluation might enable the team and organisation to learn from the experience. The team should be thanked for their efforts and then resettled, with perhaps an opportunity for the drowning of sorrows.

Evaluating the project

As discussed in Chapter 5, preparation for evaluation, and building-in data collection, reflection and review during the project will enable the organisation to assess the project's outcomes, or at least its outputs, on the basis of clear criteria and hopefully some solid evidence. It can also enable significant learning about how and why the project succeeded (or not), with potential benefit to the organisation's innovation capability. Both types of questions should be asked—that is, both outcome evaluation (the what) and process evaluation (the how and why) of project success, limitations and failure should be undertaken.

In reality, however, resistance to undertaking a formal project evaluation is common, and many of the organisations interviewed for our research indicated that they didn't do it enough, and/or did it informally. As one senior hospital manager pointed out, the bottom line is: 'You just don't get time to evaluate all the projects'. There are several reasons for this. Project reviews are sometimes let loose without specific objectives, or for 'political' motives (that is, reasons arising from power issues within the organisation). For example, an opportunity to evaluate a project that has made an unwelcome change in the role of a group of staff could become their chance to take revenge—the motives and methods of resistance (reviewed in Chapter 7) don't necessarily stop at the project's closing party. On the other hand, looking transparently at things that went wrong or need improvement, even with the best of intentions, is very confronting and tends to be avoided. And as the senior manager quoted above implies, the pressure to focus on the next goal or task undoubtedly also contributes.

Yet it is important to learn from project processes and outcomes, and some form of evaluation provides a way to crystallise the learning and formulate desired changes in approach or method. Otherwise, the short-term nature of projects provides the perfect setting for reinventing the wheel (wasting energy and time) and repeating errors (reducing the chances of success). When the project has a direct impact on patient or client care, monitoring and review are essential to assess the impact and ensure there are no adverse effects on standards or access for the client population.

Even if planning for evaluation was not done, the project plan provides an implicit basis for evaluation, and can be used for this purpose when necessary. In essence, this means that the project manager writes a simple evaluation plan based on the project's goals and objectives and uses available data as well as reflection and review activities. For example, consider the data and activities needed to complete the evaluation plan in Chapter 5 (see Table 5.6). Even after the project is complete, some of the necessary data would be available, and many of the process assessment activities could be completed as part of the final phase of the project.

Good learning can come from both informal and formal approaches. In the sections below, we address the tasks at the closing phase of the project for both approaches, starting with process evaluation.

Learning from the project experience

Reflection and learning are always happening during projects. Project managers, team members and stakeholders are engaged in figuring out how to do something new, or how to do something in a new way—so, usually, their minds are engaged at least some of the time in problem-solving and assessment of options. The challenge in process evaluation of projects is simply to stimulate and crystallise those learning and assessment activities. In the closing stages, many project participants will welcome an opportunity to engage in reflection and discussion, and are likely to be doing it in tea rooms (and possibly bars) anyway.

Some process questions can be answered with information that the project itself supplies:

- Did that approval happen on time?
- Was the report well received by the executive, sponsor and partners?
- Was the project plan modified during the course of the project?
- Did the vendor respond readily to our variance requests?
- Did the steering committee meet regularly with enough people?

Other information needs organisation to collect, and the data or information are usually qualitative in nature:

- Were the stakeholders satisfied that their views were considered and given weight?
- Were our team meetings successful in coordinating the work of the team members, and why?
- Was the communication strategy successful, and why?

- Did any changes to the plan contribute to the project's successful completion?
- Were there any difficulties that the project team encountered, and how were they overcome?

The methods of collecting the qualitative data and information generally rely on asking people the right questions in ways that enable them to be as honest and constructive as possible with the minimum possible time and effort. Face-to-face communication generally (but not always, and not for everyone) yields richer results. People think as they speak, or as they listen to others' views, and the struggle to articulate their experience helps them to understand it better and inform the evaluator more reliably. Anonymous but methodical collection of responses to questions by means other than talking (using web-based survey tools, computer-assisted 'voting' or coloured paper dots on a wall poster) can also generate information that might be hard to obtain in person.

Process evaluation towards the end of each project will be different in detail, but will generally be based on a combination of data available from the project's own documentation and some collected in person or in writing from the participants, stakeholders and intended users of the project's outcomes. Table 8.1 shows an example of the data sources in the process evaluation to be conducted in the closing phase of the surgical admissions pathway project that was introduced in Chapter 5 (Table 5.6).

Evaluating the achievement of project goals—and benefits beyond the project

Informal evaluation of the achievement of a project goal can be very simple indeed. If the goal was to implement a new information system, the question is clear: did it happen on time and on budget and to required specifications? Of course, while time and cost might be clear-cut, the question of meeting specifications is usually more complicated, and will require more effort to assess properly. There are many methods for formal evaluation of project goal achievement, as explained in Chapter 5.

As the project draws to a close, project sponsors and managers often need to look beyond the immediate concrete project goal (essentially, did we make it happen?), and consider the larger question of whether the project's results will deliver the benefits that inspired the creation of the project.

Table 8.1 Process evaluation of the surgical admissions pathway project

	Goal: To introduce a surgical admissions pathway for urgent patients straight to the receiving ward, and to test both its capacity to reduce the overall length of stay for those patients and its impact on emergency department (ED) waiting times for all patients.	
Process	**Questions**	**Data source**
Pathway development	Were staff representatives satisfied with the pathway development process?	Notes of consultations and workshops with staff representatives during the project; *notes of meeting held by an independent manager or clinical leader with staff representatives for this purpose, using questions prepared by the project team*
Stakeholder management	Were staff representatives satisfied with the project overall?	
	Was the change managed well?	Minutes of team and steering committee meetings; papers or proposals prepared by the team for the steering committee or other audiences; *notes of discussion at final steering committee meeting*
	Were other departments (including the information division) satisfied with the project process?	Minutes of meetings and other evidence of engagement with other departments; *notes of discussion held with representatives of information services, finance, bed managers and so on for this purpose*
Communication	Were stakeholders well informed about the project, its progress and the nature of changes?	Summary of all formal communication about the project with stakeholders; *notes of meetings held for evaluation purposes listed above*
Governance	Were decision-making and leadership of the project effective?	Minutes of steering committee meetings; summary of formal reports to the executive; *notes of discussion at steering committee and with executive held for this purpose; notes of other meetings held for the purpose of evaluation*
Close and handover	• Was the project closure adequate? • Was handover effective?	Summary of closure activities; notes of all questions fielded by members of the project team or the surgical division executive in the first 30 days after handover; *responses to a survey of surgical wards, ED and other departments involved in the operation*

Source: Adapted from work by Mr Jason Cloonan

Note: Data sources highlighted in italics are created specifically for the evaluation; others are existing documents or drawn from existing documents.

This question varies greatly according to the type of project. Many projects in health and community services are merely the first step, the initiation and testing of an innovation in ongoing operations or program delivery. So if the project did achieve its immediate goals—the concept was proven, the trial was successful; or the information system is in and working—the more significant question becomes 'will it deliver the benefits we seek?'. Sometimes, this question can be answered at least provisionally in the project's final report (for example, in the surgical admissions pathway project). But even in this case, the real test comes in routine operations.

These long-term questions will have been included in a good evaluation plan, but can't be answered in the closing phase of the project due to timing. Making sure that the business of answering them is identified as a future activity, and that responsibility is allocated, is one of the tasks at completion and handover.

If the benefits realisation method is being used for the project, an updated plan may need to be prepared by the project manager, perhaps with assistance from finance and information staff. It will update the original benefits realisation plan with information about progress towards achieving the intended benefits at the time of project closure; factors likely to affect success over the coming review period; and any needed changes to the method or targets (for example, ways of measuring productivity gains, or the period over which they will be realised). This updated plan should also include details as to how—and by whom—monitoring will be undertaken and final assessment made. The updated plan is then part of the formal handover of the project. A process for the approval and implementation of any recommendations for change in the benefits realisation assessment will be needed.

The same basic approach applies in the case of a project that has used a program logic model to inform the evaluation. The organisation may consider ongoing monitoring of the longer term outcomes in order to confirm (or otherwise) the effectiveness of the program. The same kind of requirements as outlined above would then apply: the measures and indicators should be confirmed or varied, and arrangements to collect the necessary data made. This (revised) plan is part of the handover, and its recommendations need to be approved and responsibility for implementation allocated.

The final report

The final report is an important element in closing a project and summing it up, either as part of acceptance and handover, or at the post-implementation review stage. Usually written by the project manager, the final report details the overall project at the point of completion and is useful as:

- an historical record of the project and what it achieved
- an opportunity for reflection on the project as a whole
- a comparison of the project at completion with the plan
- a way of informing stakeholders of the status of any outstanding issues
- a record of recommendations for future projects and strategies for sustaining the outcomes of this project
- a summary of the project evaluation, and the learning from it, with the aim of promoting enhanced capability for subsequent projects.

A good final report is structured so that the reader can quickly get a clear overview, can easily find particular information of interest, and doesn't get lost in the detail. While the size and structure of the report will depend on the nature of the project, the sections or headings shown in Figure 8.1 provide a useful starting point.

The project report should not be structured as a chronological record of the project process (the 'what I did on my holidays' approach). Rather, it should be logically structured in a way that best meets the knowledge and decision-making needs of the readers, avoids repetition, enables the reader to assess the quality and import of the information and data, and hopefully persuades readers to agree with the team's conclusions and recommendations.

The project report is usually more than a record of what happened in the project. If the report needs to help those responsible for implementing or sustaining the project's outcomes, it should focus on the practical and operational aspects of effective implementation. This would usually include the conditions under which the outcomes work well, and the minimum requirements for effective ongoing operations.

If the report needs to convince decision-makers to adopt a proposed change or sustain a project outcome, the logic of its structure should be designed to lead the reader to agree with its proposals and conclusions.

Figure 8.1 Final report template

COVER

Organisation name and logo

Name of project

Date of submission

Contents page

Executive summary
- ❑ Maximum 2–3 pages giving an overview of project background, goals, methods, outcomes, achievements, recommendations or future implications

Introduction
- ❑ Project background and purpose, the problem statement or opportunity, acknowledgements of those who made significant contributions

Project goals and methods
- ❑ Drawn from the project plan—goals, objectives, scope, strategies, program

- ❑ Budget, resourcing, sponsor, team, project organisation, committee, and so on.

Outcomes and key achievements
- ❑ Using the results of the impact evaluation

Issues
- ❑ Arising from the project but not resolved by it

Learning from the project
- ❑ A brief review of the results of the process evaluation

Recommendations and action
- ❑ Covering acceptance, handover, further monitoring and assessment of longer term outcomes or realisation of intended benefits

References
- ❑ Published sources of evidence and internal documents cited in the report

Appendices (if needed)
- ❑ Key project documents

- ❑ Details of important project data and performance indicators not included in the body of the report

One model is the 'problem–solution' structure: 'the problem is x; the possible ways of addressing it are a, b and c; we've done a lot of work to determine that b is the best method of solving the problem; and the agency should act to ensure this outcome'. If the report is needed to meet the accountability requirements of a funding body (including corporate head office), the author needs to be aware of what their expectations are, and strive to meet them.

A well-written report is a lot more convincing than one that leaves the reader to disentangle spelling errors, poor grammar and unclear meaning. Writing the contents page first is one way to focus on clear, logical structuring. Some writers find it useful to outline the report first, using dot points, others prefer to draft whole sections or paragraphs and move them around later if necessary. For most people, there is no real substitute for drafting, reading (and preferably getting others to read) and redrafting—modern word processing packages make this process much easier.

The project report may need to conform to a house style for documents. The sources of ideas and assertions in the report should be acknowledged, something that is becoming more important as agencies pursue the goals of evidence-based practice and evidence-informed decision-making. There are many acceptable referencing styles, and the agency may have a preferred style. The most important thing is to use it consistently, including for information and documents found on the internet.

If there is a wealth of important detail, it should be organised into attachments so that the data are available for those who need it (perhaps in the form of a separate volume with limited circulation). If the report has a practical use after the life of the project, it may be worthwhile to budget for a professional editor—readability can be significantly improved at a fairly modest cost.

Presentation and handover of the final report

Formal handover of the final report should also be considered. For some projects it is useful to produce a short summary document for general communication of outcomes within the organisation and among its stakeholders. Distribution of such a document also brings an opportunity to thank those who participated in workshops, interviews or consultations, and demonstrates that their input was valued.

For some projects, or some organisations, simpler documentation may be required, perhaps little more than a set of presentation slides. In any organisation, a clear, concise presentation is an effective way of communicating the project's outcomes and implications, and is a valuable adjunct to the written report. It can be worthwhile doing this well, as a good presentation can be used repeatedly to ensure that a clear, consistent message about the project is communicated to all those affected or interested in its outcomes.

Tips for effective presentations are outlined below:

- Face the audience and make eye contact. It is very tempting to focus on the overhead slides by turning around and looking at the wall—but then the audience sees the back of your head, and may think you are unprepared. When you need to check your slides, look either at a hard copy or the computer screen—then you only need to look down, rather than turning your back on the audience.
- Find a place to stand so that the audience can see both you and the screen.
- Try to relax and focus on communicating with the audience—rely on good preparation to support you while you get your message across. Connect with your audience, be enthusiastic and energetic, and dress well for the occasion.
- Show an outline slide right after the title slide. It gives the overall structure of the presentation and helps the audience know where you're taking them.
- 'Tell them what you're going to tell them, tell them, then tell them what you've told them' is an old adage for getting your message across. That is, give an outline, give your message, then sum up.
- The slides/overheads are like a skeleton—they're the structure of your presentation. All your major points should be summarised on the slides, and their relationships should be clear (for example, subpoints and correct order). They help the audience to follow your logic and know where you are heading. They also help the presenter to 'step through' the presentation.
- Put a minimum number of words on each slide. Summarise your points, don't include the full text. Each slide should have a maximum of about six lines of text, or a diagram or picture. Do not read your slides word for word, unless there's an especially good quote, or a punch line.
- The rule of thumb is one slide per minute. If you've got 15 minutes to present, you should have about 15 slides.

- The bigger the better for text size—no text should be less than 20 point, otherwise it's not readable.
- There are different opinions about colour schemes and so on. Whatever look you choose, have a strong contrast in darkness as well as colour between the background and the text—black on red, for example, is hard to read.
- Stick to time, and when you're finished, thank your audience for their attention.

Sustaining project outcomes

Lots don't achieve their outcomes, lots. Lots of them we finish and don't do anything with them if you know what I mean . . . you do the project and you finish and then nothing happens with it. A lot of that is because we're slow. Like it takes us a long time to do stuff and then you do it and you put it up for sign-off or endorsement and by then well, everyone's changed their minds and they want to do something different.

(Senior health manager)

Sustaining the project outcomes can be difficult when the project team disperses and funding is exhausted. One of the reasons for this lies in the way funding is secured and dreams are pursued. When resources are scarce, organisations sometimes enact their pursuit of better or bigger services using small dollops of project funding in order to make a start. Then they are likely to face the problem of a long journey, requiring ongoing support and resources they don't have.

The question of sustainability should be addressed at the concept stage, and dispassionate decisions are needed at that point. While there are good reasons for taking big risks very occasionally, to do so routinely is to dissipate energy, reputation, capacity and support. Our research indicates that the tendency to take on impossible or improbable challenges is still a real problem for some organisations in the sector.

There are many aspects of sustainability that the project itself cannot influence—emerging budget problems, for example. But the project method can make a difference in at least one way: by maximising the engagement of those who will be responsible for ongoing operations. If members of the future operational team are involved in the project concept, design, planning and implementation, they are more likely to be enthusiastic implementers of the outcomes.

Where the project is someone else's good idea, or is operated in a way that excludes or frustrates the receiving team, sustainability is more likely to be a rocky road. This has implications for the way in which central project units conduct their work, and emphasises again the importance of skilled engagement with stakeholders and recognition of their legitimate interests in the detailed working arrangements that the project will later seek to hand over to them.

We have also discussed the use of projects as seduction: persuading others to act by showing how a good idea can work in practice. If such a project succeeds, its existence changes the balance of probabilities (by increasing the intangible costs of denying needed funds) when ongoing resources are being divided up. Case 8.3 illustrates the point.

A successful project can also work to improve the chances of a supportive policy decision being made. It is easier for governments or health authorities to make policy supporting innovative services, or interventions in social problems, if they can point to the results of a successful trial. The success of needle exchange programs in reducing the rate of HIV infection among intravenous drug users is an example of this—the idea of handing out equipment for use in an illegal activity is otherwise hard to justify.

While there are many excellent examples of this strategy—'show it can work and then get the money (or the policy change)'—embarking on this course is a significant risk. It should be done knowingly, for very good reasons, and as an exception not the rule.

Case 8.3 Sustaining the unsustainable

An emergency response service was established with project funding in a teaching hospital. It was based in the emergency department, and mobilised resources to support emergency patients who didn't need an acute admission but couldn't go home without immediate support. It was funded as a project on the attractive theory that if it worked, it would save the hospital costs (by preventing admissions) and would therefore be self-sustaining. The project was evaluated by a major consulting firm, which found that the funding hypothesis was correct in the sense that enough admissions were avoided to cover the direct costs of providing the service. They also found that the money was not in fact available for transfer to pay for the service, because the number of admissions to the hospital was not reduced—other patients took the place of those assisted by the service.

However, the service was very popular with patients (who were able to go home with support) and with staff (who were able to move more patients through the emergency department in a timely manner). It had also been given positive coverage in the local media and was written up in an academic journal. Some of the patients became aware that the funding base was fragile and lobbied for its continuation. The end result was that the service was sustained on repeated rounds of temporary funding for at least five years.

Conclusion

Throughout this book we have emphasised the need for genuine organisational commitment to the project, for a well-developed and feasible project plan, and for adequate resources and a high-performing project team. We found that, in practice, project management in a complex industry is not just a set of competencies that can be taught from a manual but, rather, requires flexibility, understanding and good judgement.

Good judgement is not something that can be learnt from a textbook; good judgement comes from experience and a willingness to reflect and learn from that experience. As Legge et al. (2006: 15) point out, 'Where managers have real choices they cannot *know* the right answer; they have to rely on their judgment (and this means taking risks)'.

However, taking risks can be tempered through reflection on practice—what worked and what did not—and the ability to recognise the patterns or similarities in past experiences that might help to guide the project team in dealing with a current dilemma. The more we reflect and learn from our personal practice, the greater chance we have of making improved decisions when faced with complex situations.

Projects are seen as 'learning intensive organisational forms' (Disterer 2002: 512), but Disterer and others (such as Weiser & Morrison 1998) note that the boundaries between projects and the ongoing functions of the organisation can act as barriers against organisational learning from projects. This reality is seen, for example, in the fact that evaluation is rarely about improving project management practices, and that project files are stored without reference to ease of future use. Indeed, some of the lessons from project experiences are actively rejected by organisations—for example, when their implications cause discomfort because they do not fit with the espoused culture and values. Argyris (1992) describes this behaviour in terms of organisational defence mechanisms; perhaps there are 'undiscussables'—certain issues that cannot be addressed for reasons everyone may have forgotten. The organisation might also act out a number of defensive routines—for example, organising meetings that identify issues but never resolve them, instead passing them on to a proliferation of other meetings and committees (Delahaye 2000: 52).

In human services, where professional and organisational knowledge are so vital to the core functions of organisations, it is important for these barriers to be addressed. While there has been significant attention to this challenge in recent years, starting with the work of Wiig (1997) and others (Disterer 2002), recent scholarship has identified the many reasons why such efforts may not work (reviewed in Alvesson 2012). Because projects are specifically designed to be temporary efforts, the knowledge gained typically disperses with the team. There are some fairly simple steps that can be taken to counteract this tendency:

- An internal webpage or wiki could list project staff in categories of their project assignments and expertise
- In larger organisations with project support units, the role of collecting knowledge from projects could be centralised
- The project team could generate a short bulletin summarising the major learnings from the project, to be stored on the organisation's intranet or in its library
- Project team mentor roles could be fostered among experienced project managers.

When the first edition of this book was published, we expressed three hopes about the future in project management. The first was greater uptake of project approaches by organisations that face innovation and implementation challenges. Our research indicates that this hope has been at least partly realised, and the sector is now a much more sophisticated and effective user of project management.

The second was that more leaders and managers might accept the discipline of project management in their own approaches to managing change and development. We have found some progress in this area, with greater clarity and openness about goals and methods of change, willingness to support skill development, better understanding that 'the devil is in the detail', and greater respect for the real work of project teams.

The third was that using project management as a way of 'getting good ideas to work' would mean that organisations were better able to achieve their goals and meet the needs of their stakeholders. This remains the major purpose of this book, and its success is in the hands of the reader.

Summary

- Project closure is an important step in the project life cycle and needs to be actively managed. This phase includes acceptance and handover of the project outcomes and deliverables to the authorised person or group.
- Activities in project closure include a final meeting and the submission of a final report. Recognising and celebrating the efforts and achievements of those involved in the project, and planning for life after the project, are important.
- Projects can fail for a variety of reasons, and may require termination. Failing projects are sometimes allowed to drift on, and they will also need to be brought to an end. While closing a failed project can be difficult, once failure is clear, closure should be prompt and decisive.
- Evaluation of projects in the health and community services sector is important, and can be formal or informal. The outcomes or outputs, as well as the processes, should be evaluated, so that those involved can know both what worked well and what didn't, and why.

- Program logic and benefits realisation assessment are two useful methods for evaluating the project and establishing the basis for longer term assessment of outcomes.
- Sustaining the outcomes of a project can be difficult, but is more likely where members of the future operational team are involved in the project concept, design, planning and implementation.

Readings and resources

Centers for Disease Control and Prevention: http://www.cdc.gov/eval/resources/index.htm

South Australian Community Health Research Unit, Flinders University, 'Planning and Evaluation Wizard': http://som.flinders.edu.au/FUSA/SACHRU/PEW/Index.htm

Project Management Knowhow, 'Project termination' (managing the early termination of a project): http://www.project-management-knowhow.com/project_termination.html

Project templates

Figure 4.1 Project proposal template

Name of project:

Project sponsor: **Proposer:**

1. **Background to the project:** [Briefly explain the context and the problem or opportunity that gives rise to the project]

2. **Goals and objectives:** [What is the project aiming to achieve?]

3. **Rationale:** [Why should these goals be pursued through a project?]

4. **Scope:** [Briefly state the boundaries of the project. What is included and what is excluded?]

5. **Deliverables:** [What will this project produce?]

6. **Stakeholders:** [Who has power and influence? Who will be directly affected by the project? What are their concerns likely to be?]

7. **Timeframe and resourcing estimates:** [What is the likely duration of the project? Likely types and amounts of resources (labour and non-labour) required? What is the likely source of funding?]

8. **Risks and key assumptions:** [Identify all known major risks the project faces, and outline the major assumptions that may affect the project's viability or success]

Sign-off: ——————————————————————————————————

Proposer: ———————————————— Sponsor: ————————————————

Date: ———————————————— Date: ————————————————

Figure 6.5 Business case template

Executive summary
- ❏ A concise summary (ideally on two pages) of the content of the document, including all recommendations. It should read as a 'stand alone' document, and should not introduce any material not found in the body of the report.

Sign-off sheet
- ❏ For recording project sponsors' and proponents' signatures, committing them to act on the business case, or recording their support.

Current situation
- ❏ A statement of the background and current context with relevant facts and judgements backed up with evidence (expressed in numbers where possible).

Future state
- ❏ The intended, predicted or desired future situation or environment. That is, the realisation of goals and strategies; the future role delineation; risk profile; and service models and so on. Any assumptions should be clearly set out and supported with relevant data or other evidence.

Policy issues
- ❏ The broad policy, political, legislative and organisational constraints within which the business case must fit. For example, government policies, social justice considerations, legislative requirements, accreditation.

Strategic alignment
- ❏ Alignment of this initiative with organisational/government strategic goals.

Gap/needs analysis
- ❏ A statement of the problems, gaps or needs that the project seeks to address, supported with relevant data and analysis.

Options for action
- ❏ All feasible options to address the problems or gaps within the policy constraints. Each option, including the 'base case' or 'do nothing' option, should be described in enough detail to establish workable alternative courses of action. Each option must be capable of standing alone.

Analysis of options
- ❏ Qualitative and quantitative analysis including income and expenditure streams; sources of funds for capital and recurrent costs; economic analyses (such as cost utility); risk analysis; volume of outputs or services; strategic considerations; and timing. The analysis of each facet should conclude with a definitive result or solution, since these results will be used for comparison and selection of a preferred option.

Evaluation and selection of preferred option
- ❏ Based on the results of the steps above and a clear statement of the criteria and process, the preferred option is identified (and usually also appears in the executive summary).

Recommendations
- ❏ The preferred option is presented in the form of a decision or action for decision-makers to endorse or decline. Any needed information about decision-making and approval processes and the management of perceptions should be included.

Implementation plan
- ❏ Specifies the team or individual responsible for implementation, and outlines the main components of the project plan.

Appendices (if needed)
- ❏ Material referred to but not included in the business case. For example, members of the project team; additional financial or service data and analysis; demographic/population profiles; equipment lists; and references.

Figure 7.3 Change request template

1. Project information			
Submission date:		Reference:	
Initiating party:			
Project description:			

2. Change scope	
Description of change required:	
Justification:	

3. Project impacts	
Schedule/time:	
Cost:	
Other:	
Priority:	
On approval by all parties, the required change/s will be subject to quotation/confirmation of cost	

4. Project status and currency	
Implementation details:	
Current phase:	
Implementation completion date:	

5. Approvals and signatures				
Project manager:		Approved	Yes/No	Date:
Project sponsor:		Approved	Yes/No	Date:

Figure 7.5 Project status report template

Project status report for period ending: / /

1. Project summary

Project name	
Sponsor	
Approved budget	
Actual start date	
Forecast end date	
Project manager	
Current phase	*i.e. initiation, planning, implementation, closure, review*
Current status	*Green, amber or red**

* Indicator definitions: Green = [as planned], Amber = [signs of trouble], Red = [in trouble]

2. Progress

Project phases and activities	% Complete	Planned start date	Actual start date	Planned end date	Actual end date

Key accomplishments last period:

Upcoming tasks for this period:

3. Project financials <Financial year>

Cost item	Approved budget $	Actual $	Forecast overrun $	Comment

4. Key project issues

Issue no.	Issue	Management

5. Key project risks

Risk no.	Risk	Mitigation

6. Change requests

Change request	Change description	Impact

7. Key communications/Planned events

Date	Description

Figure 8.1 Final report template

COVER
Organisation name and logo
Name of project
Date of submission

Contents page

Executive summary
- ❑ Maximum 2–3 pages giving an overview of project background, goals, methods, outcomes, achievements, recommendations or future implications

Introduction
- ❑ Project background and purpose, the problem statement or opportunity, acknowledgements of those who made significant contributions

Project goals and methods
- ❑ Drawn from the project plan—goals, objectives, scope, strategies, program

- ❑ Budget, resourcing, sponsor, team, project organisation, committee, and so on.

Outcomes and key achievements
- ❑ Using the results of the impact evaluation

Issues
- ❑ Arising from the project but not resolved by it

Learning from the project
- ❑ A brief review of the results of the process evaluation

Recommendations and action
- ❑ Covering acceptance, handover, further monitoring and assessment of longer term outcomes or realisation of intended benefits

References
- ❑ Published sources of evidence and internal documents cited in the report

Appendices (if needed)
- ❑ Key project documents

- ❑ Details of important project data and performance indicators not included in the body of the report

Project management courses in Australia

ACT	Australian National University	• Short: Management Framework for Business Projects • Graduate Certificate in Management (Project Management)
NSW	University of Technology Sydney	• Short: Continuing Professional Education • Graduate Certificate in Project Management • Master of Project Management
NSW	University of Wollongong	• Master of Project Management
NT	Charles Darwin University	• Certificate IV in Project Management • Diploma of Project Management
QLD	Bond University	• Postgraduate Diploma in Project Management • Graduate Certificate in Project Management • Master of Project Management
QLD	Queensland University of Technology	• Master of Project Management
QLD	University of Queensland	• Graduate Certificate in Project Management • Graduate Diploma in Project Management • Master of Project Management
SA	University of Adelaide	• Master of Applied Project Management
SA	University of South Australia	• Graduate Certificate in Project Management • Graduate Diploma in Project Management • Master of Project Management

VIC	Victoria University	• Master of Project Management
VIC	Swinburne University	• Diploma of Project Management
WA	Curtin University of Technology	• Short: Project Management Fundamentals • Graduate Certificate in Project Management • Graduate Diploma in Project Management • Master of Science (Project Management)
WA	Edith Cowan University	• Graduate Certificate in Project Management • Graduate Diploma in Project Management • Master of Project Management
Other	TAFE	• Cert IV in Project Management
Other	Australian Institute of Project Management (AIPM)	• Project management short course • Project management certification
Other	Blue Maple	• Prince 2 • PMBOK® • Short courses in project management
Other	eCertIT	• Project Manager Professional certification • PMBOK®
Other	HiLogic Project Management	• Prince 2 training • Short courses in project management
Other	PM Training Online	• Short courses in project management
Other	PM-Partners Group	• Prince 2 training • Short courses in project management

Other	ProJ Study	• Prince 2 training • Short courses in project management
Other	Project Management	• Project management certification and training • Prince 2 • PMBOK®
Other	Seek Learning	• Project Management Institute (PMI®) certified courses • PMBOK®

References

Alsene, E. (1998). 'Internal changes and project management structures within enterprises'. *International Journal of Project Management*, 17(6), 367–76

Alvesson, M. (2012). 'A stupidity-based theory of organizations'. *Journal of Management Studies* accepted article. doi: 10.1111/j.1467-6486.2012.01072.x

Andersen, E. S., Birchall, D., Jessen, S. A., & Money, A. H. (2006). 'Exploring project success'. *Baltic Journal of Management*, 1(2), 127–47.

Argyris, C. (1992). *On Organizational Learning*. Cambridge, Mass: Blackwell.

Assudani, R., & Kloppenborg, T. J. (2010). 'Managing stakeholders for project management success: an emergent model of stakeholders'. *Journal of General Management*, 35(3), 67–80.

Atkinson, R. (1999). 'Project management: cost, time and quality, two best guesses and a phenomenon, it's time to accept other criteria'. *International Journal of Project Management*, 17, 337–42.

Aveyard, H. (2010). *Doing a literature review in health and social care: A Practical Guide*. London: Open University Press.

Belassi, W., & Tukel, O. (1996). 'A new framework for determining critical success/failure factors in projects'. *International Journal of Project Management*, 14(3), 141–51.

Belout, A., & Gauvreau, C. (2004). 'Factors influencing project success: the impact of human resource management'. *International Journal of Project Management*, 22(1), 1–11.

Bradshaw, J. R. (1972a). 'The concept of social need'. *New Society*, 496, 640–43.

Bradshaw, J. R. (1972b). 'The taxonomy of social need'. In G. McLachlan (ed), *Problems and Progress in Medical Care* (pp.71–84). Oxford: Oxford University Press.

Brown, K., Waterhouse, J., & Flynn, C. (2003). 'Change management practices: Is a hybrid model a better alternative for public sector agencies?'. *International Journal of Public Sector Management*, 16(3), 230–41.

Burke, R. (2003). *Project management: planning and control techniques*. West Sussex: John Wiley & Sons.

Carter, R., & Harris, A. (1999). 'Evaluation of health services'. In G. Mooney & R. Scotton (eds), *Economics and Australian Health Policy* (pp.154–71). Sydney: Allen & Unwin.

Case, R. (1998). 'The structure of high-performing project management organisations'. *Drug Information Journal*, 32, 577–607.

Central Computer and Telecommunications Agency (CCTA) (1997). *PRINCE 2: An Outline*. Norwich: TSO.

Chen, H. (2010). 'The bottom-up approach to integrative validity: A new perspective for program evaluation'. *Evaluation and Program Planning*, 33(3), 205–14. doi:10.1016/j.evalprogplan.2009.10.002

Chen, H. L. (2011). 'Predictors of project performance and the likelihood of project success'. *Journal of International Management Studies*, 6(2), 101–10.

Cleland, D. I., & Gareis, R. (2006). *Global project management handbook*. New York: McGraw-Hill Professional.

Cleland, D. I., & King, W. R. (2008). *Project management handbook* (2nd edn). West Sussex: John Wiley & Sons.

Consumers Health Forum of Australia (2008). *Engaging Consumers*. Canberra: CHFA. Retrieved from: https://www.chf.org.au/pdfs/cns/cns-489-engaging-consumers.pdf

Cookson, R. (2008.) 'Evidence-based policy making in health care: what it is and what it isn't'. *Journal of Health Service Research and Policy*, 13(3), 118–21.

Courtney, M., & Briggs, D. (2004). *Health care financial management*. Sydney: Elsevier.

Day, G. E., Visawasm, G., & Briggs, D. (2004). 'The budget and financial control'. In M. Courtney & D. Briggs (eds), *Health care financial management* (pp. 173–84). Sydney: Elsevier.

DeFilippi, R. J. (2001). 'Introduction: Project-based learning, reflective practices and learning outcomes'. *Management Learning* 32(1), 5–10.

Delahaye, B. (2000). *Human Resource Development: Principles and practice*. Brisbane: John Wiley & Sons.

Department of Health and Ageing (2002). *Supporting innovation in patient care: NDHP*. Canberra: Commonwealth of Australia.

Department of Industry, Science and Resources (2000). 'Shaping Australia's future innovations—framework paper'. Canberra: Commonwealth of Australia.

DeSimone, L., Porter, A., Garet, M., Yoon, K. S., & Birman, B. (2002). 'Effects of professional development on teachers' instruction: Results from a three-year longitudinal study'. *Educational Evaluation and Policy Analysis*, 24(81), 81–112.

Disterer, G. (2002). 'Management of project knowledge and experiences'. *Journal of Knowledge Management*, 6(5), 512–20.

Dobie, C. (2007). *A handbook of project management: A complete guide for beginners to professionals*. Sydney: Allen & Unwin.

Dobson, M. (1996). *Practical Project Management: The secrets of managing any project on time and on budget*. Mission, Kansas: Skillpath Publications.

Drummond, M. F., Sculpher, M. J., Torrance, G. W., O'Brien, B. J., & Stoddard, G. L. (2005). *Methods for the economic evaluation of health care programmes* (3rd edn). New York: Oxford University Press.

Dunphy, D., & Stace, D. (2001). *Beyond the boundaries: leading and recreating the successful enterprise* (2nd edn). Sydney: McGraw-Hill.

Dwyer, J. (2004). 'Australian health system restructuring—what problem is being solved?'. *Australia and New Zealand Health Policy*, 1(6). doi:10.1186/1743-8462-1-6

Eagar, K., Garrett, P., & Lin, V. (2001). *Health planning: Australian perspectives*. Sydney: Allen & Unwin.

Edmondson, A. (1999). 'Psychological safety and learning behavior in work teams'. *Administrative Science Quarterly*; Jun 1999; 44, 2; ABI/INFORM Global pp. 350–83.

Egan, G. (1994). *Working the Shadow Side: A guide to positive behind the scenes management*. San Francisco: Jossey Bass.

Fink, A. (2010). *Conducting research literature reviews: from the Internet to paper* (3rd edn). Los Angeles: SAGE.

Finkler, S. (1994). *Essentials of cost accounting for health care organisations*. Maryland: Aspen Publishers.

Fortune, J., & White, D. (2006). 'Framing of project critical success factors by a system model'. *International Journal of Project Management*, 24(1), 53–65.

Funnell, S. (1997). 'Program logic: An adaptable tool for designing and evaluating programs'. *Evaluation News and Commentary*, 6, 5–17.

Gido, J., & Clements, J. (1999). *Successful Project Management*. Ohio: International Thomson Publishing.

Goldratt, E. M. (1994). *It's not luck*. Great Barrington, Mass: North River Press.

Gormley, K. K., & Verdejo, T. (2000). 'A systems approach—budgeting for the 21st century: turning challenges into triumphs'. *Nursing Administration Quarterly*, 24 (4), 51–9.

Hamilton, R. L. (1964). *Study of methods for evaluation of the PERT/Cost Management System*. Massachusetts: The Mitre Corporation.

Hartley, S. (2009). *Project Management: principles, processes and practice* (2nd edn). Frenchs Forest: Pearson Education Australia.

Haugan, G. T. (2003). *The Work Breakdown Structure in Government Contracting*. Vienna: Management Concepts.

Hawe, P., Degeling, D., & Hall, J. (1990). *Evaluating health promotion, a health worker's guide*. Sydney: Maclennan & Petty.

Hayes, H. B. (2002). 'Using earned-value analysis to better manage projects'. *Pharmaceutical Technology*, 26(2): 80–4.

Haynes, M. (1994). *Project Management: From idea to implementation*. UK: Crisp Publications.

Head, B.W. (2010). 'Reconsidering evidence-based policy: key issues and challenges'. *Policy and Society: an interdisciplinary Journal of Policy Research*, 29(2), 77–94.

Healy, P. (1997). *Project management: Getting the job done on time and on budget*. Melbourne: Butterworth, Heinemann.

Hibbard, J. (2003). 'Engaging Health Care Consumers to Improve the Quality of Care'. *Medical Care,* 41(1, Supplement), 161–70.

Hill, G. M. (2010). *The complete project management methodology and toolkit*. Roca Raton: CRC Press.

Hindle, D. (1997). *Financial management in health services*. Sydney: MacLennan & Petty.

HRM Advice. (2008). 'The organisational climate'. Retrieved from http://hrmadvice. com/hrmadvice/hr-strategy/the-organizational-climate.html

Ika, L. A. (2009). 'Project success as a topic in project management journals'. *Project Management Journal*, 40(4), 6–19.

Johnson, J. (2010). *Get a GRPI on Six Sigma teams*. Ridgefield: ISixSigma. http://www. isixsigma.com/implementation/getting-started-implementation/get-grpi-six-sigma-teams/

Kahn, E. F. (1982). 'Critical themes in the study of change'. In P. S. Goodman & associates (eds), *Change in Organisations* (pp. 409–29). San Francisco: Jossey Bass.

Keil, M., Mann, J., & Rai, A., (2000). 'Why software projects escalate: an empirical analysis and test of four theoretical models'. *MIS Quarterly*, 24(4), 631–64.

Kerzner, H. (2009). *Project management: A systems approach to planning, scheduling, and controlling* (10th edn). Hoboken: John Wiley & Sons.

Kliem, R. L. (2007). *Effective communications for project management*. Portland: Auerbach Publications.

Kliem, R. L., Ludin, I. S., & Robertson, K. (1997). *Project Management Methodology: A practical guide for the next millennium*. New York: Marcel Dekker Inc.

Kloppenborg, T. J. (2009). *Contemporary project management: organize, plan, perform*. Mason, USA: South-Western Cengage Learning.

Kotter, J. & Schlesinger, L. (1979). 'Choosing strategies for change', *Harvard Business Review*, March–April, 106–14.

Kovacevic, M., Odeley, O., Sietsema, W. K., Schwarz, K. M., & Torchio, C. R. (2001). 'Financial concepts to conducting and managing clinical trials within budget'. *Drug Information Journal*, 35(3), 1031–38.

Kovner, A., & Rundall, T. G. (2006). 'Evidence based management reconsidered'. *Frontiers of Health Services Management*, 22(3), 3–22.

Lao Tse (1963). *Tao te ching: The way of virtue* (trans by Patrick M. Byrne). New York: SquareOne Classics.

Latham, G. P., & Locke, E. A. (1979). 'Goal-setting: A motivational technique that works'. *Organizational Dynamics*, 8(2), 68–80.

Lavis, J., Davies, H., Oxman, A., Denis, J., Golden-Biddle, K., & Ferlie, E. (2005). 'Towards systematic reviews that inform health care management and policy-making'. *Journal of Health Services Research & Policy*, 10(Supplement 1), 35–48.

Leggat, S., Balding, C., & Anderson, J. (2011). 'Empowering health-care managers in Australia: an action learning approach'. *Health Services Management Research*, 24, 196–202. doi: 10.1258/hsmr.2011.011012

Leggat, S., & Dwyer, J. (2003). 'Factors supporting high performance in health care organisations: A review of the literature'. Melbourne: National Institute of Clinical Studies.

Legge, D., Stanton, P., & Smyth, A. (2006). 'Learning management (and managing your own learning)', (pp. 1–24), in M. Harris, *Managing Health Services: Concepts and practice* (2nd edn). Sydney: Mosby Elsevier.

Levasseur, R. E. (2010). 'People skills: ensuring project success—a change management perspective'. *Interfaces*, 40(2), 159–62.

Lewin, K. (1958). 'Group decisions and social change'. In E. Maccoby (ed), *Readings in Social Psychology* (pp. 197–211). New York: Holt, Rinehart & Winston.

Liang, Z. (2011). *Program development and evaluation subject lecture note*. Melbourne: La Trobe University.

Liang, Z., Howard, P. F., & Rasa, J. (2011). 'Evidence-informed managerial decision-making—what evidence counts? (part one)'. *Asia Pacific Journal of Health Management*, 6(1), 23–9.

Liang, Z., & Howard, P. F. (2011). 'Evidence-informed managerial decision-making—what evidence counts? (part two)'. *Asia Pacific Journal of Health Management*, 6(2), 12–21.

Lientz, B., & Rea, K. (1998). *Project Management for the 21st Century* (2nd edn). San Diego: Academic Press.

Lock, D. (2007). *The essentials of project management* (9th edn). Burlington USA: Gower Publishing Company.

Longest, B. B. (2004). *Managing health programs and projects*. San Francisco: Jossey–Bass.

McCawley, P. F. (1997). *The Logic Model for Program Planning and Evaluation*. Moscow: University of Idaho Extension.

McElroy, W. (1996). 'Implementing strategic change through projects'. *International Journal of Project Management* 14(6), 325–29.

McLaughlin, J., & Jordan, G. (1999). 'Logic models: a tool for telling your program's performance story'. *Evaluation and Program Planning*, 22, 65–72.

Martin, V., & Henderson, E. (2001). *Managing in Health and Social Care*. London: Routledge.

Martin, V. (2002). *Managing projects in health and social care*. New York: Routledge.

Martini, A. (2006). *Community participation in government and private sector planning: A case study of health and telecommunications planning for rural and remote Western Australia.* (Doctoral Dissertation, Murdoch University, Western Australia). Retrieved from http://researchrepository.murdoch.edu.au/184/2/02Whole.pdf

Maylor, H. (1996). *Project Management*. London: Pitman Publishing.

Meredith, J. R., & Mantel, S. J. (2009). *Project management: a managerial approach* (7th edn). New York: John Wiley & Sons.

Mintzberg, H. (1991). 'Ideology and the missionary organisation'. In H. Mintzberg & B. Quinn (eds), *The Strategy Process: Concepts, contexts, cases* (pp. 352–58). Englewood Cliffs, New Jersey: Prentice-Hall.

Mishra, P., Dangayach, G. S., & Mittal, M. L. (2011). 'An empirical study on identification of critical success factors in project based organisations'. *Global Business and Management Research: An international Journal*, 3(3&4), 356–68.

Morteza, S. & Kamyar, K. (2009). 'Generic project success and project management success criteria and factors: Literature review and survey'. *World Scientific and Engineering Academy and Society Transactions on business and economics* 6(8), 456–68.

Nadler, D., & Tushman, M. (1997). 'Implementing new designs: managing organizational change', in M. Tushman & P. Anderson (eds), *Managing Strategic Innovation and Change: A collection of readings*. New York: Oxford University Press.

NHS Institute for Innovation and Improvement (2008). *Quality and Service Improvement Tools: Benefits Realisation*. Retrieved from http://www.institute.nhs.uk/quality_and_service_improvement_tools/quality_and_service_improvement_tools/benefits_realisation.html

Nilsson, S., Baigi, A., Marklund, B., & Frjdlund, B. (2001). 'The prevalence of the use of androgenic anabolic steroids by adolescents in a county of Sweden'. *European Journal of Public Health*, 11(2), 195–7.

NSW Government (2009). *Benefits realisation plan*. Retrieved from http://services.nsw.gov.au/sites/default/files/Benefits%20Realisation%20Plan%202011_0.doc

Oisen, R. P. (1971). 'Can project management be defined?'. *Project Management Quarterly*, 2(1), 12–14.

O'Kelly, S. W., & Maxwell, R. (2001). 'Implementing clinical governance. Medical training should include project management'. *British Medical Journal*, 323(7315), 753.

Overton, R. (2001). *Business planning: Writing a business plan.* Sydney: Angus and Robertson.

Parliamentary Office of Science and Technology (2003). *Government IT projects*, Report 200, London: POST. Retrieved from: http://www.parliament.uk/documents/post/pr200.pdf

Partington, D. (1996). 'The project management of organizational change'. *International Journal of Project Management*, 14(1), 13–21.

Patton, M. Q. (1990). *Qualitative Evaluation and Research Methods.* Thousand Oaks, CA: Sage Publications.

Pawson, R., & Tilley, N. (1997). *Realistic Evaluation.* London: Sage Publications.

Perkins, R., Petrie, K., & Alley, P. (1997). 'Health service reform: the perceptions of medical specialists in Australia (NSW), the United Kingdom and New Zealand'. *Medical Journal of Australia*, 167:201–204.

Pinto, J. K. (2000). 'Understanding the role of politics in successful project management', *International Journal of Project Management*, 18(2): 85–91.

Pinto, J. K., & Slevin, D. P. (1988). 'Critical success factors across the project life cycle'. *Project Management Journal*, 19(3), 67–75.

PRINCE2® (2009). *PRINCE2 basics*, PRINCE2, London. Retrieved from www.prince2-2009basics.com

Project Management Institute (PMI). (2008). *A Guide to the Project Management Body of Knowledge* (4th edn) (PMBOK® Guide). Newtown Square, Pennsylvania: PMI.

Proudlove, N.C., Gordon, K., & Boaden, R. (2003). 'Can good bed management solve the overcrowding in accident and emergency departments?'. *Emergency Medicine Journal*, 20, 149–55.

Queensland Treasury (1997). *Managing for Outcomes: Output Specifications Guidelines.* Brisbane: Queensland Treasury.

Revans, R. W. (1998). *ABC of Action Learning.* London: Lemos & Crane.

Roberts, P. (2011). *Effective project management: identify and manage risk—plan and budget—keep projects under control.* London: Kogan Page.

Rosacker, K., Zuckweiler, K. M., & Buelow, J. R. (2010). 'An empirical evaluation of hospital project implementation success'. *Academy of Health Care Management Journal*, 6(1), 37–53.

Rosenau, M. D. J. (1998). *Successful Project Management.* New York: John Wiley & Sons.

Roughley, A. (2009). *Developing and using program logic in natural resource management: user guide.* Canberra: Commonwealth of Australia.

Royse, D., Thyer, B. A., Padgett, D. K., & Logan, T. K. (2006). *Program evaluations: an introduction* (4th edn). Belmont, CA: Thomson Brooks/Cole.

Royse, D., Station-Tindall, M., Badger, K., & Webster, J. M. (2009). *Needs assessment pocket guide to social work research methods.* New York: Oxford University Press.

Rubin, H. J., & Rubin, I. (1992). *Community Organizing and Development* (2nd edn). New York: Macmillan.

Rummler, C. A., & Brache, A. P. (1995). *Improving Performance: How to manage the white space on the organisation chart.* San Francisco: Jossey-Bass.

Sa Couto, J. (2008). 'Project management can help to reduce costs and improve quality in health care services'. *Journal of Evaluation in Clinical Practice*, 14(1):48–52.

Shenhar, A. J., & Dvir, D. (2007). *Reinventing project management*. Boston: Harvard Business School Press.

Shore, B., 2008. 'Systematic Biases and Culture in Project Failures'. *Project Management Journal* 39(4), 5–16.

Shortell, S. M. (2006). 'Promoting evidence-based management'. *Frontiers of Health Services Management*, 22(3), 23–9.

Skinner, Q., & Price, R. (eds) (1990). *Machiavelli: The Prince*. Sydney: Cambridge University Press.

South Australian Community Health Research Unit (SACHRU) (2012). *Planning and evaluation wizard*. South Australia: Flinders University.

Stephenson, T. (1985). *Management: A Political Activity*. Basingstoke: Macmillan.

Taylor, A. G., & Rafai, S. (2003). 'Strategic budgeting: a case study and proposed framework'. *Management Accounting Quarterly*, 5(1), 1–10.

Taylor-Powell, E., Jones, L., & Henert, E. (2003). 'Enhancing Program Performance with Logic Models'. University of Wisconsin'. Retrieved from: http://www.uwex.edu/ces/pdande/evaluation/pdf/lmcourseall.pdf

Turner, J. R. (2007). *Gower handbook of project management* (4th edn). Burlington: Gower Publishing Limited.

Van Horne, J. (1998). *Financial management and policy* (11th edn). New Jersey: Prentice Hall.

Verzuh, E. (2011). *The fast forward MBA in project management* (4th edn). Hoboken, New Jersey: John Wiley & Sons.

Victorian Ombudsman (2011). *Investigation into ICT-enabled projects*. Melbourne: Victorian Ombudsman.

Vos, T., Carter, R., Barendregt, J., Mihalopoulos, C., Veerman, J. L. et al. (2010). *Assessing Cost-Effectiveness in Prevention (ACE–Prevention): Final Report*. Brisbane: University of Queensland & Melbourne: Deakin University.

Wadsworth, Y. (2010). *Building in Research and Evaluation: Human inquiry for living systems*. Sydney: Allen & Unwin.

Webster, G. (1999). *Managing Projects at Work*. Hampshire, UK: Gower Publishing Ltd.

Weiser, M., & Morrison, J. (1998). 'Project memory: Information management for project teams'. *Journal of Management Information Systems*. 14(4), 149–66.

Westerveld, E. (2003). 'The project excellence model: linking success criteria and critical success factors'. *International Journal of Project Management*, 21, 411–18.

Westland, J. (2006). *The project management life cycle: a complete step-by-step methodology for initiating, planning, executing & closing a project successfully*. London: Kogan Page.

White, D., & Fortune, J. (2002). 'Current practice in project management: An empirical study'. *International Journal of Project Management*, 20(1), 1–11.

Wiig, K. M. (1997). 'Knowledge Management: An Introduction and Perspective'. *Journal of Knowledge Management*, 1(1), 6–14.

Wilson, G., & Wright, M. (1993). *Evaluation Framework*. Melbourne: CDIH.

Index